THE HIGH INSTENSITY WORKOUT

DR JOHN BABRAJ AND DR ROSS LORIMER

THE HIGH INTENSITY WORKOUT

THE FAST TRACK TO FITNESS AND HEALTH

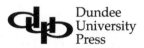

Dundee
University
Press

First published in Great Britain in 2012 by
Dundee University Press
University of Dundee
Dundee
DD1 4HN

ISBN 9781845861476

British Library Cataloguing-in-Publication Data
A catalogue record for this book is available on request
from the British Library

Typeset by Zebedee Design
Printed by Bell & Bain Ltd., Glasgow
Cover by Sandra Friesen

ACKNOWLEDGEMENTS

I would like to acknowledge Prof. Jamie Timmons and Dr. Niels Vollaard, without them I may never have started to research high intensity exercise. I would also like to express my heart felt gratitude to Allison Fannin, her support and proof reading of this book made it possible.

CONTENTS

1 HIGH-INTENSITY TRAINING AND PERFORMANCE   **9**

2 HIGH-INTENSITY TRAINING AND HEALTH   **27**

3 THE MENTAL ELEMENTS OF HIGH-INTENSITY TRAINING   **51**

4 PRACTICAL ASPECTS OF HIGH-INTENSITY TRAINING   **70**

5 MYTHS AND MISCONCEPTIONS ABOUT EXERCISE   **96**

1

HIGH-INTENSITY TRAINING AND PERFORMANCE

When we talk about performance we mean your body's ability to carry out a set task. In a sporting context, performance means your body's ability to carry out a sporting task such as running or sprinting possibly combined with a skill task such as dribbling a ball. It goes without saying that different people will have different sporting performance levels. For one person just completing a 5km run is a good performance whereas someone else will be setting out to win the 5km race. What both these athletes tend to have in common is a desire to carry out the run as fast as they can, and as long as they believe they have done this then they will be happy with their performance. One of the key factors in determining whether you are just seeking to finish or are challenging to win is the level of training that you do. To get the best performance you need to train to make your body adapt to allow you to be the best that you can be. High-intensity training is one way of getting the best performance that you can, getting physiological adaptations quickly with an extremely time-efficient training regime.

WHAT IS HIGH-INTENSITY TRAINING?

High-intensity training is brief periods of repeated bursts of all-out exercise interspersed with longer periods of recovery. The intensity of the training session associated with high-intensity training can be controlled in a variety of ways, such as the intensity of the sprint, the duration of the sprint or the number of sprints performed. The duration and number of intervals performed will determine the total time commitment for the training session but most typical high-intensity training protocols last no more than fifteen minutes in total with between one and three minutes of actual exercise. Due to the adaptations that high-intensity training produces in the body, these will be the most effective fifteen minutes of exercise you have ever had.

PERFORMANCE IMPROVEMENTS

Performance improvements occur following all training to start with. You get fitter for the sport that you are training for, whether it is a long-distance run or a triathlon. The level of the improvements that occurs with a training programme depends on the stress that you put on your body during training. If you stay within your comfort zone then you will struggle to improve your performance beyond its current level. Effective training will alter how your body fuels the exercise; this is known as exercise metabolism. The two main metabolic pathways (metabolic pathways are chemical reactions in the cells, controlled by enzymes, which regulate cell behaviour) that are altered are the *aerobic* and *anaerobic* energy production systems.

AEROBIC METABOLIC PATHWAY

The term *aerobic* means with oxygen. Aerobic metabolism is the use of fuel sources in the presence of sufficient oxygen. During exercise there are different fuels your body can access to allow your body to move. Blood glucose is a major source of energy during exercise. During exercise there is a 700% increase in glucose being taken out of the blood and entering skeletal muscle. The blood glucose is provided by the liver breaking down its stored glucose (known as glycogen), or making new glucose molecules from lactate, pyruvate and amino acids. There is also a 300% increase in fat taken out of the blood and entering skeletal muscle. The blood fats are provided by the fat tissue breaking down its stored fat (known as triglyceride) or from circulating triglycerides made in the liver. The skeletal muscles also have their own fat and glycogen stores which can be accessed to fuel the exercise and about 50% of the fat that is used during exercise comes from the skeletal muscles' own fat stores. During moderate-intensity continuous exercise we use these fuels mainly via the aerobic pathway.

Aerobic metabolism requires special processing units within the cells known as mitochondria. Mitochondria are unique in that they have their own genetic footprint separate from the cell itself. Use of mitochondria is the most efficient way that the body can produce adenosine triphosphate (the energy currency of the body) through the tri-carboxylic acid metabolic pathway. This produces approximately 12 times more adenosine triphosphate from glucose than is released by the anaerobic pathway. The aerobic metabolic pathway is the only way that the body can use fat as a fuel source. The fat is converted to a smaller molecule before passing into the mitochondria where, in the presence of glucose, it is converted into adenosine triphosphate through the tri-carboxylic acid metabolic pathway. The tri-carboxylic pathway is controlled by enzymes, proteins within the cell that speed up metabolic reactions.

Delivery of oxygen to the cells is controlled by the heart. The faster the heart beats, the greater the speed of delivery of blood to the cells. Oxygen is carried around the body in the bloodstream to where it is needed, so the greater the delivery of blood then the greater the delivery of oxygen. Your ability to fuel the exercise aerobically is not limited by the amount of oxygen in your bloodstream (you only use a small proportion of the oxygen that you breathe in); it is the ability of the body to actually use the oxygen fast enough that limits your ability to fuel your exercise aerobically. When you struggle to fuel your exercise aerobically then the anaerobic pathway will be used but it can only fuel the exercise for a limited period resulting in a decrease in performance.

ANAEROBIC METABOLIC PATHWAY

The term *anaerobic* means without oxygen. However, we are never in a situation where no oxygen is available so we never truly fuel the skeletal muscle 100% by the anaerobic pathway. In human metabolism anaerobic means the use of carbohydrate with insufficient oxygen. The only fuel that can be used anaerobically is glucose. When insufficient oxygen is available, glucose from the blood or from glycogen is broken down and converted to lactate, with the release of adenosine triphosphate. The amount of adenosine triphosphate created is relatively low (about 8% of that created when glycogen is used aerobically). The lactate will either be used to fuel further the skeletal muscle movement or it will be exported out of the skeletal muscle and into the blood where it can be used elsewhere as fuel, for example, the heart or brain. When anaerobic metabolism is used there is a large amount of glycogen utilised. This means that the skeletal muscle fuel reserves are rapidly lost, and therefore anaerobic metabolism can only fuel exercise for a very short period of time. Anaerobic metabolism will be used when the heart cannot deliver enough oxygen-rich blood to the working skeletal muscle. Even if you are running or cycling at a constant low speed you will use anaerobic metabolism at the start of the exercise as the heart has not yet responded to the demands for energy that the skeletal muscle is making.

Unlike aerobic metabolism, there is no need for special processing units within the cell for anaerobic metabolism. Anaerobic metabolism takes place within the cytoplasm of the cell (the cytoplasm is the fluid that fills the cells where all the contents of the cell are found). Even though there is no special processing unit, anaerobic metabolism is, like aerobic metabolism, controlled by enzymes.

ENDURANCE PERFORMANCE

Endurance exercise is defined as exercise that is performed over an extended period of time and endurance performance refers to your body's ability to perform exercise over an extended period of time. When training to improve endurance performance you are seeking to extend the length of time that you can perform an exercise for, or the speed at which you can cover a set distance. Both of these measures can be used by sports scientists to determine somebody's endurance performance. The most commonly used test to assess endurance performance capacity is a VO_2 max test. This tests your body's ability to deliver oxygen during increasingly higher-intensity exercise. The higher your VO_2 max the greater your endurance capability is but not necessarily your endurance performance. Elite marathon runners Grete Waitz and Derek Clayton have VO_2 max values of 73 and 69 $ml.kg^{-1}.min^{-1}$ respectively yet Derek Clayton's personal best time in the marathon was 15 minutes faster than Grete Waitz. Oxygen delivery is clearly not the only physiological variable that determines endurance performance. There are three main physiological variables that account for approximately 80% of your endurance performance:

The skeletal muscles' aerobic metabolism

Skeletal muscle aerobic metabolic capacity is directly related to the numbers of mitochondria in the skeletal muscle. The greater the number of mitochondria available the more fuel can be utilised aerobically. The inability of skeletal muscles to consume oxygen has been recognised for over 100 years as a limit to exercise performance.

Blood lactate concentration during exercise

The ability of the body to maintain a low blood lactate concentration at any particular exercise intensity is a reliable measure of endurance performance. Blood lactate concentration is a balance between skeletal muscle lactate production and whole body lactate use. If the mitochondrial capacity (that is, aerobic capacity) of the skeletal muscle is small then lactate will be produced much more quickly as the skeletal muscle utilises anaerobic metabolism to fuel the exercise.

Oxygen delivery to the skeletal muscles

Oxygen delivery is controlled by how fast and strong your heart beats, blood flow through the circulatory system and the oxygen-carrying capacity of the blood. The oxygen-carrying capacity of blood is determined by the number of red blood cells present. Red blood cells make a protein called haemoglobin and oxygen is carried in the blood attached to haemoglobin. Therefore the more red blood cells you have, the more haemoglobin you will have to increase the amount of oxygen that can be carried. This is often one area that elite athletes will seek to abuse by illegally increasing red blood cell production by injecting erythropoietin (EPO) as they seek to improve their endurance performance. EPO is a hormone and its role in the body is to increase the production of new red blood cells.

IMPROVEMENTS IN ENDURANCE PERFORMANCE FOLLOWING ENDURANCE AND HIGH-INTENSITY TRAINING

As we have said, the most commonly used test to determine endurance capacity is a VO_2 max test. The figure shows a typical VO_2-intensity curve during increasing exercise intensity. As the exercise gets harder you breathe in more oxygen until you can no longer increase the supply of oxygen. This point in the curve is known as your VO_2 max. Following six weeks of endurance training you normally see between a 5 and 10% improvement in VO_2 max. If you look at the figure, you can see that there is a shift in the VO_2-intensity curve to the right. Following high-intensity training the change in VO_2 max varies depending on the intensity of the sprint training. In studies that have used fewer high-intensity workout sessions (six sessions over two weeks) no significant change in VO_2 max has been noted but other studies utilising more workout sessions (14 sessions over two weeks) have reported increases of 12% in VO_2 max. This suggests that there may be a minimum number of high-intensity workout sessions required to see improvements in VO_2 max. However, VO_2 max has limits that are set by your genetics so if you are already training it is difficult to see improvements in this test.

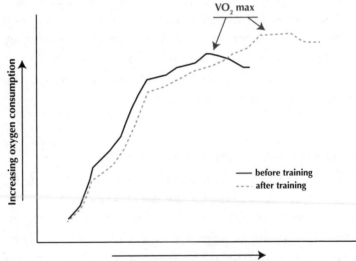

A more sport-specific measure of endurance performance is the time trial test. This test requires the participant to run or cycle as fast as possible for a set distance.

Improvements in endurance performance are easier to detect in these tests due to the genetic limitations to improvements in VO_2 max. Two weeks of endurance training will increase time trial performance by 7%; two weeks of high-intensity training will increase it by 10%, but the number of workout sessions required for the high-intensity training is only six compared to ten sessions of endurance training. In longer-term comparison studies similar improvements in performance are seen with 18 sessions of high-intensity training compared to 30 sessions of endurance training. So, while the improvements are similar, high-intensity training requires less training time (10 minutes for high-intensity training compared to 90 minutes for endurance training). When 12 sessions of high-intensity training have been added into somebody's endurance training (with a reduction of 15% in miles covered per week), time trial performance was reduced by 1.5 minutes compared to no change when high-intensity sessions were not added. This demonstrates that most people who train for endurance performance eventually reach a point where they cannot continue to improve performance using traditional endurance training as they are already spending a large amount of their time clocking up miles.

ANAEROBIC EXERCISE PERFORMANCE

Anaerobic performance can be described as your body's ability to respond rapidly to exercise demands when insufficient oxygen is available, that is, during a sprint or at the start of or at the end of fatiguing exercise. When training to improve anaerobic performance you are seeking to generate as much power in the skeletal muscles as quickly as possible or to resist fatigue for as long as possible after VO_2 max has occurred. The most commonly used test to explore this is a cycle-based test which requires an all-out effort for 30 seconds against a set resistance. The factors that determine anaerobic performance are still not fully known but two physiological measures have been suggested to be important for your anaerobic exercise performance.

How much blood lactate increases during the short-duration exercise bout

Lactate is made during anaerobic metabolism, and when you are exercising at a high intensity the amount of lactate produced by the skeletal muscles is greater than the amount of lactate being used by the body. This leads to blood lactate concentration increasing. The greater blood lactate concentration is, the better your anaerobic exercise performance will be.

How much power you can produce when blood lactate levels have increased to 10 millimoles per litre of blood

Blood lactate concentration is normally between 1 and 2 millimoles per litre of blood. The amount of power that your skeletal muscles can produce during short-duration exercise is directly related to the anaerobic utilisation of glycogen. As blood lactate concentration rises you are using the fuel in the skeletal muscles. The better adapted your skeletal muscles are to anaerobic exercise, the greater the power you can produce when this fuel is being depleted.

IMPROVEMENTS IN ANAEROBIC EXERCISE PERFORMANCE FOLLOWING ENDURANCE AND HIGH-INTENSITY TRAINING

The most commonly used test for anaerobic exercise performance is the 30-second sprint test. Endurance-trained athletes such as long-distance runners have been shown to have a poor power production in this test. Their power production was no better than somebody who was untrained. The blood lactate rise after this 30-second test in endurance-trained athletes is approximately 10 millimoles per litre compared to 15 millimoles per litre in sprint-trained athletes. Following high-intensity training, anaerobic exercise performance increases, with power production increasing between 10 and 20% following six training sessions.

When looking at the ability of a person to fuel exercise above the body's aerobic capacity, that is, above the exercise intensity where VO_2 max occurs, both endurance and high-intensity training have been shown to increase the length of time that you can perform this exercise intensity for. The metabolic systems used at this intensity of exercise are the same in both endurance and high-intensity trained individuals. Following six high-intensity workout sessions over two weeks, the time that people work at above VO_2 max was increased by 10%, whereas only a 4% increase is seen after 13 weeks of endurance training. For both these training exercise methods, this shows a better ability to use the anaerobic fuel metabolism, however, the size of the improvement is much bigger following high-intensity training compared to endurance training.

HOW DOES HIGH-INTENSITY TRAINING IMPROVE PERFORMANCE?

There are a number of different adaptations that occur following high-intensity training that will lead to improvements in performance. Which ones together or alone are the most important is not known but when we consider the physiological determinants of endurance and anaerobic exercise performance then there are a number of adaptations that result in improved performance.

SKELETAL MUSCLE MITOCHONDRIAL ADAPTATIONS

Skeletal muscle mitochondria are the energy centres for aerobic metabolism. They are vital in converting glucose and fat into energy (adenosine triphosphate) and require a sufficient supply of oxygen to do this. This requirement for oxygen in the mitochondria is the reason why we have to breathe. Sports performance demands an extremely efficient aerobic energy system to deliver optimal performance. Even in short duration sprint events lasting only 30 seconds aerobic metabolism plays a crucial role in fueling the skeletal muscle. Therefore, one key to developing performance is to enhance the number and efficiency of skeletal muscle mitochondria. Adaptation of skeletal muscle mitochondria is probably one of the most important adaptations to training and will enable you to perform closer to your true potential.

How does high-intensity training regulate skeletal muscle mitochondria?

An improvement in aerobic metabolism and mitochondrial

density in skeletal muscle is often seen following traditional endurance training. It has been demonstrated that skeletal muscle mitochondrial density does not increase continuously with exercise duration. Exercise durations longer than 60 minutes at constant intensities do not significantly increase mitochondrial enzyme densities above that seen with constant-intensity exercise of a shorter duration.

A consistent finding in high-intensity training studies is an increased mitochondrial density and enzyme activity in skeletal muscle. High-intensity workouts of between two and six weeks duration, consisting of repeated 30-second cycle sprints, increase the aerobic metabolism capacity of the skeletal muscle. There is an increase in the amount of protein of a key regulator of aerobic metabolism (PGC1) in skeletal muscle. This occurs through an increase in mitochondrial protein synthesis. When this protein is artificially over-expressed in animals it results in a dramatic shift of skeletal muscle fibre type, moving to a more aerobic type of fibre, with an increase in mitochondrial density. There is a 30% greater increase in expression of this protein following high-intensity training compared to endurance training.

There are other mitochondrial protein adaptations to high-intensity training. High-intensity workouts of between two and six weeks' duration, consisting of repeated 30-second cycle sprints, increase the total amount and activity of the protein that is rate limiting for aerobic metabolism (COX4). Rate limiting means that it is the activity level of this enzyme that determines how fast the reaction can proceed at. COX4 is a mitochondrial enzyme involved in electron transfer on the mitochondrial inner membrane. Other skeletal muscle mitochondrial proteins are also increased following two weeks of high-intensity training. The activity of the enzymes involved in the tri-carboxylic acid cycle, the site of adenosine triphosphate production, are increased following high-intensity training. This means the skeletal muscle is able to process fuel in the presence of oxygen faster and more efficiently. All this suggests that improved skeletal muscle mitochondrial density and aerobic capacity occurs rapidly and to a greater extent than traditional endurance exercise following high-intensity training. The major signal necessary to promote mitochondrial adaptations is the reduction in adenosine triphosphate and phosphocreatine, which happens to a greater extent following high-intensity training than traditional endurance training.

ALTERED LACTATE METABOLISM
Lactate used to be thought of as a waste product produced during exercise. However, lactate is anything but a waste product. It is an exceptionally important fuel during exercise (used by skeletal muscle, heart, brain and other tissues) and the more efficient your use of lactate during exercise the stronger your overall performance will be.

How is lactate made?
Lactate is produced when insufficient oxygen is available during the breakdown of glucose to make adenosine triphosphate (this process is known as anaerobic glycolysis). During glycolysis when sufficient oxygen is available (aerobic glycolysis), the glucose is broken down; producing pyruvate that then enters the tri-carboxylic acid cycle to produce adenosine triphosphate. When insufficient

oxygen is available then the pyruvate molecules produced during glycolysis are converted into lactate. The lactate can then be moved out of the exercising skeletal muscle and transported to other tissues, such as non-working skeletal muscle, heart or brain, where lactate can be used as an important fuel source. When the amount of lactate being produced by the working skeletal muscles is greater than the amount of lactate that can be used by the rest of the body, then blood lactate accumulation occurs.

How does high-intensity training regulate lactate metabolism?

One of the ways that high-intensity training is thought to improve performance is by improving whole body lactate utilisation. When we do exercise of increasing intensity the amount of lactate in the blood starts to increase once the intensity is high enough. This point where blood lactate starts to build up is known as the lactate threshold. Following two weeks of high-intensity training, there is a rightward shift of the blood lactate curve during increasing-intensity exercise. This can be seen in the figure which shows that there is an increase in work intensity required to cause blood lactate concentrations to increase. The reason for this improvement is in part due to improved use of the available lactate. Within the working skeletal muscle there is less lactate accumulation following two weeks of high-intensity training. This decrease in lactate accumulation in the skeletal muscle during increasing-intensity exercise could be due to a decreased rate of glycogenolysis (the breakdown of glycogen), increased clearance of lactate and uptake elsewhere or an increased use of pyruvate in oxidative metabolism. Following high-intensity training there is an increase in skeletal muscles' ability to transport lactate through increased amounts of the protein required to allow lactate into or out of the skeletal muscle cells. It has been shown that the more of this transporter protein you have, the greater the uptake of lactate into that skeletal muscle cell will be. This suggests that there is an improved ability of non-working skeletal muscles to take an increased amount of lactate out of the blood following high-intensity training. This will result in a lower blood lactate accumulation during exercise. There is an extremely strong relationship between the absolute exercise intensity required to raise blood lactate concentration and endurance performance.

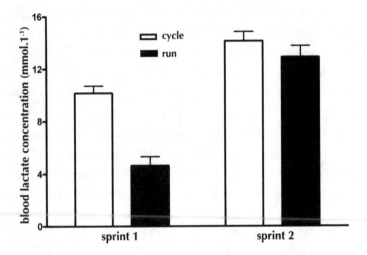

CHANGES IN THE CARDIOVASCULAR SYSTEM

The cardiovascular system includes your heart, blood vessels and blood. Its function is to deliver oxygen, nutrients and hormones around the body. Your heart forces the oxygen-rich blood through the arteries to the different tissues. Once the blood reaches the tissues the oxygen is released and waste products such as carbon dioxide are picked up. The oxygen-depleted blood then travels back to the heart through the veins. Once the oxygen-depleted blood has returned to the heart it is pumped to the lungs where it releases carbon dioxide and picks up oxygen again before being returned to the heart and the whole cycle can start again.

Long-term exercise training has been shown to produce a variety of different changes in the blood vessels and heart, leading to the heart being able to pump the blood more efficiently around the body. Following high-intensity training and endurance training there are similar changes in the extent of cardiac growth. However, only high-intensity training, and not endurance training, improves heart function. After high-intensity training, there is improved mitochondrial activity in the heart muscle (allowing the heart to fuel itself aerobically), increased efficiency of the heart (with a lower oxygen demand at the same exercise intensity) and changed fuel use (with a greater increased use of carbohydrates). These adaptations to high-intensity training will allow the heart to sustain its output at maximal intensities of exercise and therefore improve endurance performance.

Exercise economy

The oxygen required to be taken up by the body at specific exercise intensities is known as exercise economy. A better exercise economy, that is, a lower oxygen demand at a given intensity, is advantageous for an endurance athlete. This is because the body is better able to meet the demands of the exercise with less demand for fuel which allows you to exercise for longer or to exercise at a faster pace. Very few studies have shown improvements in exercise economy following short-term exercise training. Six weeks of endurance training has been shown to improve running economy by 3%. Following two weeks of high-intensity training, cycling economy is improved by approximately 8%. This improvement in exercise economy following high-intensity training is much bigger than is seen with endurance training and occurs much more quickly. The improvements seen in exercise economy are directly related to improvements in skeletal muscle mitochondrial density, and as seen above high-intensity training produces bigger adaptations in mitochondrial enzyme content and activity than endurance training.

CONCLUSION

Your performance is directly related to the training you undertake. Variation in the workload of the training sessions and oxygen uptake during the training sessions, rather than the total time spent performing the training sessions or how much energy you use during the training sessions, are the key factors which increase the skeletal muscles' ability to utilise fuel in the aerobic pathway. Likewise, your skeletal muscles' adaptation to the training to allow it to utilise the anaerobic fuel pathway is much bigger when the workloads of the training sessions are high. High-intensity training is the optimal training protocol to maximise the adaptations in the skeletal muscle. The adaptations in the skeletal muscle lead to big improvements in both endurance and anaerobic exercise performance.

2

HIGH-INTENSITY TRAINING AND HEALTH

Health is a complicated concept. It has traditionally meant the absence of disease or illness but now has a much more holistic meaning that encompasses physical, mental and social wellbeing. Being physically active has been shown to have a positive impact on all of these aspects: reducing disease risk, enhancing mood and expanding social inclusion. One of the biggest risks to health is being unfit. Being overweight and unfit increases your risk of ill health by more than 200% compared to somebody who is lean and fit. However, if you are overweight and are fit then your risk of ill health is only 10% more than somebody who is lean and fit. Instead of 'you are what you eat' it should be 'you are what you do'.

Inactivity and a lack of fitness are directly linked to two of the biggest diseases in modern society: type 2 diabetes and heart disease. In a number of research studies, starting and maintaining an exercise programme has been shown to be more effective than drugs at lowering your risk of developing either of these two diseases. It has also been shown that making somebody, who is otherwise fit and healthy, inactive produces changes in the body which are similar to those seen in people who have been diagnosed with type 2 diabetes. The amount of time you spend sitting and watching television is related to your risk for type 2 diabetes and heart disease. That is why type 2 diabetes and heart disease are commonly called lifestyle diseases. It is the choices you make in terms of your diet and activity that are the biggest determining factors in whether or not you will get them. This chapter will explore the science behind improvements in physical wellbeing when you do high-intensity training specifically in relation to these two diseases.

WHAT IS TYPE 2 DIABETES?

Type 2 diabetes is a disease that makes your body unable to remove excessive glucose from the blood. When we eat a meal the carbohydrates in the meal are digested and broken down into glucose. The glucose then goes into the blood stream to be stored in the skeletal muscle and liver as glycogen and in fat tissue as glycerol. The removal of glucose from the blood after eating is controlled by the hormone insulin. When blood glucose levels are increased there is a corresponding increase in blood insulin levels. Insulin binds to a protein on the outside of the skeletal muscle cells (known as a receptor protein) and this triggers a change in activity of the proteins involved in allowing glucose to enter the skeletal muscle. The end result is that more of the glucose transporter protein is moved from inside the skeletal muscle cells to the skeletal muscle cells' outside shell allowing more glucose into the skeletal muscle. You might think of insulin acting as the key to the door of the skeletal muscle, opening the door to allow glucose into the muscle cells. This removal of glucose from blood after eating takes approximately two hours.

In people with type 2 diabetes, when the meal is eaten the blood glucose is not removed quickly even though there has been an increase in blood insulin. More and more insulin is released as the body reacts to the raised blood glucose levels. This phenomenon is known as insulin resistance. As type 2 diabetes progresses, the body can no longer continue releasing the high levels of insulin required to overcome insulin resistance and lower the blood glucose. This leads to a constantly excessive blood glucose level, which means all the tissues in the body are continuously bathed in this energy-rich blood. Some of the tissues can alter how much glucose they take from the blood but others cannot. Long-term tissue damage is caused in those tissues that cannot change how much blood glucose that they take up.

WHY IS EXERCISE IMPORTANT IF I HAVE TYPE 2 DIABETES OR I DO NOT WANT TO GET IT?

For a long time it has been known that exercise such as weight training, running or cycling are effective ways of managing the symptoms of type 2 diabetes and lowering the risk of getting type 2 diabetes.

TYPE 2 DIABETES AND EXERCISE

Exercise has been shown to lower blood glucose levels. When you exercise there is a big demand for glucose from the skeletal muscle, almost a 700% increase in skeletal muscle glucose uptake from the blood, to provide the energy required for the body to move. Unlike when we eat, this skeletal muscle glucose uptake is not controlled by the hormone insulin but by different factors such as nitric oxide. The elevated blood glucose levels seen in people with type 2 diabetes will be reduced closer to normal levels. The harder the exercise, the bigger the reduction in blood glucose will be, that is, you will lower blood glucose more running for one hour compared to walking for the same time. This means that somebody with type 2 diabetes who exercises regularly will have better management of their blood glucose and this will significantly lower their risk of the associated complications. As well as lowering blood glucose levels, exercise also improves insulin sensitivity in people with type 2 diabetes. Insulin sensitivity is a measure of how responsive the body is to insulin – a comparison between blood glucose levels and blood insulin levels following the drinking of a glucose solution. The quicker you lower your blood glucose levels and the less insulin that is required to do this, the more sensitive your body is to insulin. Exercise training changes the properties of the proteins that respond to insulin making them able to react much better. This means that when somebody with type 2 diabetes eats a meal the blood glucose levels are lowered much more quickly. However, the effects of the exercise bout are short-lived, lasting about 24 hours, after which the blood glucose levels rise again. To continue the improvements, exercise has to be carried out routinely.

TYPE 2 DIABETES RISK AND EXERCISE

Your risk of getting type 2 diabetes is directly related to your lifestyle, that is, the more active you are, the lower your risk is for getting type 2 diabetes. It has been shown that in people who are at a high risk of getting type 2 diabetes traditional exercise programmes are a much more effective treatment than the leading pharmaceutical intervention. Exercise lowers your risk over three years by approximately 60% compared to a decrease of approximately 30% through pharmaceutical intervention.

People without type 2 diabetes do not normally have raised blood glucose levels but exercise still acts to improve insulin sensitivity. Any improvement in insulin sensitivity will lower your risk of getting type 2 diabetes. Traditional exercise programmes, such as weight training, running or cycling, have all been shown to improve insulin sensitivity 24 hours after the last exercise session. However, the improvements in insulin sensitivity do not last and will return to pre-training levels within 72 hours of the last exercise session. Therefore, to maintain a reduced risk you need to continue exercising routinely.

HIGH-INTENSITY TRAINING AND IMPROVEMENTS IN INSULIN SENSITIVITY

High-intensity training is an exceptionally time-efficient way to improve insulin sensitivity. Following just six high-intensity training sessions, insulin sensitivity has been shown to be improved by 25% in inactive people. This is a much bigger increase in insulin sensitivity in just two weeks compared to traditional exercise programmes lasting 8 to 12 weeks. With traditional training programmes you do not normally see improvements in insulin sensitivity in two weeks. The improvement in insulin sensitivity was accompanied by a reduction of 10% in blood glucose levels following drinking 75g of glucose. This is remarkable when you consider that in similar studies using traditional training the level of blood glucose following drinking 75g of glucose does not change after training. What high-intensity training and traditional training do is to lower the amount of insulin required to get the 75g of glucose out of the blood stream compared to before somebody starts to train. However, the high-intensity training required 30% less insulin whereas traditional training generally requires 10 to 15% less insulin. Not only is the size of the improvements bigger with high-intensity training, the total time commitment per training session is much lower (20 minutes, of which only two to three minutes was exercise, compared to anywhere between 40 to 60 minutes of exercise per session for traditional training programmes). This means that high-intensity training sessions can be more easily fitted around your lifestyle.

The other major difference between high-intensity training and traditional training is how long the health adaptations last. In traditional training the improvements of insulin sensitivity are seen only 24 hours after the last training session. In high-intensity training improvements in insulin sensitivity are seen 72 hours after the last training session. This means that the health adaptations to high-intensity training are much longer lasting and occur much quicker than traditional training. So what does high-intensity training do to the body to produce such big adaptations?

WHY DOES HIGH-INTENSITY TRAINING YIELD SUCH BIG IMPROVEMENTS IN INSULIN SENSITIVITY?

With high-intensity training there are three potential mechanisms that regulate the improvement in insulin sensitivity. It is highly likely that improvements are due to an additive effect of all three mechanisms, rather than one or the other.

Glycogen turnover

Glycogen is the storage form of glucose. Glycogen is a chain of glucose molecules joined together with the chains of glucose branching out from a central point. This structure allows glycogen to store glucose efficiently and provide the greatest energy return as glucose molecules can be removed from many different branches at the same time. Glycogen turnover is the process whereby glycogen is broken down and used for energy and then remade after you provide the body with carbohydrates.

When you eat a meal you provide your body with an excess of energy (in the form of glucose, amino acids and fat) that it does not need to use straight away. These energy sources are removed from the blood and stored for when you have a period of high-energy demand (that is, when you are exercising). Glucose can be stored in skeletal muscle, liver or fat tissue. This process is controlled by insulin and the most important tissue, in terms of the amount of glucose taken up and stored, is the skeletal muscle. The glycogen content of liver accounts for about 8% of the tissue mass and about 2% for skeletal muscle mass. However, the liver weighs approximately 1.5kg, and stores 120g of glycogen, whereas skeletal muscle weighs approximately 14kg, and stores 280g of glycogen. This makes skeletal muscle the major site of glycogen storage. Once the glucose is inside the skeletal muscle cells it still needs to be processed into glycogen. This is a multi-stage process under the control of proteins called enzymes. Insulin increases the activity of some of these enzymes, accelerating the time taken for glucose to be added to the glycogen chain. In the liver, insulin does not increase glucose transport but it accelerates the time taken for glucose to join the glycogen chain.

When there is an increase in energy demand, that is, when you exercise, then some of the glycogen in the skeletal muscles and liver are broken down to meet the energy demands. The amount of glycogen broken down depends on how much energy your body needs. In skeletal muscle the glycosyl (glucose) units released from glycogen enter the energy system of the skeletal muscle to produce adenosine triphosphate. In contrast, the liver converts the glycosyl (glucose) units back to glucose which means it can be transported back out of the liver cells and into the bloodstream to provide energy where it is needed in the body. Once the energy demand has decreased then glycogen will be remade for future use.

Why is glycogen turnover important for insulin sensitivity?

Skeletal muscle glycogen is a bank of energy that the skeletal muscle will use when excessive demands are placed on it. If the skeletal muscle is not breaking the stored glycogen down then there is no need for the skeletal muscle to take glucose out of the blood to remake it. The glycogen will expand and take up more space in the skeletal muscle. Any glucose that is taken up into the skeletal muscle will increase the branching of the glycogen. This branching of glycogen makes it more difficult to break it down for fuel when needed. This growth in glycogen will lead to impairment in the passage of glucose out of the blood stream as the skeletal muscle does not need it nor has the room to store it. Rather than being stored in the skeletal muscle the excess blood glucose is instead taken up by the fat tissue and converted to glycerol and stored as fat. Increased fat mass leads to the release of fat hormones known as adipokines, which can act to impair skeletal muscle glucose uptake. As well as adipokine release there is increased fat around tissues, in particular liver and skeletal muscle, which impairs the insulin-controlled metabolic pathways. This means that you can still produce the key (insulin) to the door but when you push against the door it only opens a little, leading to impaired insulin sensitivity.

How does high-intensity training regulate glycogen turnover?

When we exercise we place increased demands on the skeletal muscle, which if the intensity is high enough will result in glycogen use. However, with low-intensity exercise of a moderate duration very little skeletal muscle glycogen or fat is used. Instead, the energy demands of the exercise are adequately met by energy supplied from the liver. It is only during prolonged exercise of a moderate intensity or during higher-intensity exercise that skeletal muscle substantially accesses its glycogen stores. Skeletal muscle never utilises all of its glycogen stores during exercise, with approximately 30% of the stored glycogen remaining unused in the skeletal muscle. Due to the nature of high-intensity exercise there is a large demand placed on the skeletal muscle for rapid movement, and this is provided predominantly by the skeletal muscles' own energy stores: adenosine triphosphate, phosphocreatine and glycogen. Two 30-second sprints will use all of the skeletal muscles' glycogen stores that can be accessed. In a typical 30-second protocol (see chapter 4), four sprints are normally performed with the skeletal muscle struggling to produce the same power in sprints three and four. In the shorter duration 6-second protocol (see chapter 4), by the end of ten sprints you will have used all the accessible skeletal muscle glycogen stores. After the high-intensity training session the skeletal muscle has a markedly increased demand for glucose to allow it to replenish its glycogen stores. Over a two-week high-intensity training programme this translates into increased skeletal muscle glycogen stores known as supercompensation, as the skeletal muscle adapts to the stresses placed on it and ensures there is enough fuel available for subsequent high-intensity training sessions. This supercompensation of glycogen is driven by the increase in the glucose transporter protein in the skeletal muscle. When insulin then binds to its receptor protein on the skeletal muscle cell there is more transporter protein, which could be moved to the skeletal muscles' outside shell and this increases the amount of glucose that can be taken into the skeletal muscle for the same amount of insulin. Therefore, insulin sensitivity is improved.

Protein turnover

Proteins are the functional control centre of the body. They provide the structural framework for cells and tissues, catalyse reactions within the cells and regulate communication between different parts of your body. Your genes need to be converted into proteins to make you into you. This is a two-step process where the genes are read and make messenger RNA, which is then converted into the protein. Protein turnover is the term given to the constant making and breaking down of proteins within the body. Different tissues have different rates of protein turnover; but a typical 70kg man would make and break approximately 300g of protein every day. Approximately 20% of your basal energy use goes into protein turnover.

Once a protein is made it becomes exposed to the stresses and strains of the body. This will change the biochemical properties of the protein and alter how well it performs its specific role within the cell. Protein turnover is a natural process during which these older damaged proteins are removed and new undamaged proteins are made ensuring that the cells can continue to function optimally. Protein turnover is stimulated by a variety of different factors.

When we wake up in the morning and have not eaten for hours we are in a state of fast and are in a situation of protein deficit. This means that we are breaking down more proteins than we are making. When we eat, the pathways that make proteins are switched on and this results in an increase in protein production. At the same time the pathways involved in the breakdown of proteins are switched off, allowing the cells to regain protein. As well as being affected by fasting and eating the turnover of proteins is also regulated by our activity levels. When we exercise, our skeletal muscles utilise energy to fuel the exercise rather than to make proteins – thus the rate of protein synthesis slows down because this process uses a lot of energy that is required to fuel the exercise. During exercise the rate that the proteins are broken down increases, which provides amino acids to be used as fuel. When we stop exercising then there is a large increase in the rate that proteins are made. This can persist for up to 48 hours after the exercise. However, over the course of 24 hours there is a balance between the rate that proteins are made at and the rate that they are broken down, which means the protein content of the cells remains constant.

Why is it important in improvements in insulin sensitivity?

Insulin-regulated uptake of glucose into the skeletal muscle is controlled by a protein-signalling cascade. You might think of this as a domino rally: when one protein gets activated it leads to another being activated and so on until you reach the end of the rally (in this case glucose transporter protein moving to the outside shell of the cell). If this cascade is working correctly then you get increased glucose taken up into the skeletal muscle cells when insulin binds to the receptor protein and initiates that domino rally. However, as the proteins age, their ability to respond normally to insulin changes, due to exposure to different chemicals which alter their structure, and if this were allowed to happen then less glucose would be taken up into the skeletal muscle cells. Therefore, you need to constantly break down damaged proteins to ensure that the insulin response of the skeletal muscle is maintained.

How does high-intensity training regulate this?

Exercise controls the rate that we make proteins in two ways. In the immediate aftermath of exercise the rate that messenger RNA is converted into protein is increased. The longer-term adaptation to the exercise stress is an increased conversion of the genes into messenger RNA and then into protein. High-intensity training is no different in how it controls protein turnover. However, it has been shown that two weeks of high-intensity training increases the total amount of the glucose transporter protein in skeletal muscle. As there is more glucose transporter protein then the skeletal muscle's response to insulin will be magnified, leading to more glucose being taken up by the skeletal muscle. In longer-term high-intensity training studies the same increase in glucose transporter protein has been shown. However, after stopping the high-intensity training the amount of glucose transporter gradually declines, but it is still much higher six weeks after training than it was before the training. This means that even six weeks after doing high-intensity training people were more insulin-sensitive than before they started the training.

Fat metabolism

Like glycogen and protein, fat is constantly being made and broken down. The processes involved in this are collectively known as fat metabolism. If you eat more food than you need, based on what you do, then the body will store the excess energy as fat. Genetically this allows us to survive during periods of food shortage. However, we no longer live in a hunter-gatherer society; if we are not active then we will continue to store more and more energy as fat. Fat can be stored in the adipose tissue (fat tissue) or in deposits close to the mitochondria, the power station of cells needed for producing energy, in skeletal muscle cells. When we exercise we utilise the fat from the skeletal muscle stores and from the adipose tissue in the mitochondria to help fuel the exercise session. The skeletal muscle has a huge demand for energy during exercise and fatty acids will be taken out of the blood to be used for energy. Once we eat we replace these stores again, preparing the energy systems for the next challenge. As we train, the mitochondria of the cells become much more efficient at generating energy from our fuel sources due to the increased protein turnover that occurs with exercise. This means more fatty acids can be removed from the blood even at rest, which lowers the level of fat in the blood. Traditional exercise programmes that have been designed to promote fat loss focus on low-intensity, long-duration exercise, as it is believed that we use more fat at this intensity.

What role does fat have in insulin sensitivity?

Excessive fat deposits in skeletal muscle have a negative effect on insulin sensitivity. The more fat that is deposited in and around the skeletal muscle, the worse your insulin sensitivity will be. The fat deposits interfere with the protein-signalling pathway that responds to insulin. When insulin binds to its receptor on the outer shell of the muscle cell, the signalling pathway is not activated in the same way meaning less glucose transporter will move to the outer shell and therefore less glucose will enter the skeletal muscle. If we again imagine insulin as a key then it can still go into the lock but the door is more difficult to open and more insulin is required to force the door open. Paradoxically, elite athletes also have a high level of fat deposits in and around the skeletal muscle but they are found to be exceptionally insulin-sensitive. The major difference between somebody who is insulin-sensitive and an elite athlete is that the elite athlete will use these fat stores to help fuel their training and competition. Somebody who is insulin-insensitive is likely to be physically inactive, meaning these fat deposits will not be getting used and will then interact with the proteins in the skeletal muscle to change their structure. This change in the structure means that they can no longer respond as well to insulin.

Excessive fat will also be deposited around the liver. Just like with the skeletal muscle this interferes with the insulin response in the liver. Normally in response to insulin binding to its receptor on the liver cells the rate that glycogen is made at increases and the liver pathways that release glucose into the blood are switched off. However, with excessive fat around the liver this does not happen, which means that the liver still releases glucose into blood. If you consider that when you eat a meal the carbohydrates are broken down to glucose, if your liver does not respond to insulin normally then blood glucose levels are raised even higher. Your skeletal muscles will not be taking the glucose out of the blood quickly which means that you will have a prolonged raised glucose level. This is dangerous and over a long period of time can lead to blindness, kidney failure and heart disease.

How does high-intensity training regulate fat metabolism?

When you do a single high-intensity exercise session the rate that you break down fat stores from your fat tissue and skeletal muscle fat deposits increases, causing an increase in available fatty acids. These fatty acids can be taken up into skeletal muscle and converted by the mitochondria into adenosine triphosphate. As the skeletal muscle is exercising it requires a large amount of fuel which means all the fuel reserves will be used to some extent. The length of the high-intensity sprint or the number of repetitions in a training session will determine the magnitude of fat use during the session. Two of the hormones that control fat breakdown, adrenaline and noradrenaline, are elevated by as much as 1450% following a high-intensity training session. The size of this response is much bigger than is seen with steady exercise such as jogging or cycling.

When you have been involved in high-intensity training specific adaptations occur in the skeletal muscle. The most important of these regarding fat metabolism is the increased number of mitochondria found in skeletal muscle. This means that the skeletal muscle has a greater capacity to use fatty acids as a fuel source. As well as increased mitochondria in the skeletal muscle there is also increased mitochondrial protein activity. This is consistently found across all high-intensity training interventions. When performing traditional exercise after high-intensity training there is a 36% increase in the amount of fat used to fuel the exercise. The increased fat use is because there is an increased activity of the protein that is believed to limit the rate that fatty acids can be used by the mitochondria. Even at rest there is a lower amount of circulating free fatty acids after two weeks of high-intensity training. This is important as it lowers your risk of heart disease.

In longer-duration, high-intensity training these skeletal muscle adaptations result in a reduction of fat mass of between 10 and 40%. Particularly important for insulin sensitivity and type 2 diabetes risk is the amount of fat stored around your abdomen. The reduction in fat around the abdomen following high-intensity training is approximately 8% in 12 weeks. This is a consistently bigger loss in abdomen fat mass than is seen with traditional continuous exercise. There is also a bigger loss of fat that is stored under the skin of about 10 to 15%. Again this is much bigger than you find with traditional continuous exercise. This loss of fat mass is associated with a significant increase in insulin sensitivity.

HEART DISEASE

Heart disease is a generic term used to discuss a variety of different diseases associated with the heart and blood vessels. Together the heart, blood vessels and blood are given the term the cardiovascular system. When people talk about heart disease they often mean just coronary heart disease (angina and heart attack) but there are many more diseases associated with the cardiovascular system such as stroke, heart failure and hypertension. Approximately a third of all deaths in the UK are due to heart disease, with coronary heart disease being the biggest killer. Like type 2 diabetes, an individual's lifestyle plays a big part in whether they develop cardiovascular disease.

WHAT IS THE CARDIOVASCULAR SYSTEM?

The cardiovascular system is your heart, blood vessels and blood. Its function is to deliver oxygen, nutrients and hormones around the body. The heart is the central tissue of the cardiovascular system. It pumps oxygen-rich blood through the arteries around the body to the different tissues. Once the blood reaches the tissues the oxygen is released and waste products such as carbon dioxide are picked up. The oxygen-depleted blood then travels back to the heart through the veins. Once the oxygen-depleted blood has returned to the heart it is pumped to the lungs where it releases carbon dioxide and picks up oxygen again before being returned to the heart where the whole cycle can start again. On average your heart beats 100,000 times per day to ensure adequate delivery of oxygen around the body. As well as delivering oxygen, this circulation of blood ensures that when you eat, the nutrients that are released are taken to peripheral tissue for storage or other tissues that require energy. Also the blood is the major way that different tissues talk to each other through the release of hormones. For example, the raised blood glucose levels that occur when you eat are detected in the pancreas, which triggers the pancreas to release insulin into the blood. The insulin then travels around the body in the bloodstream until it can interact with the appropriate tissues and promote glucose uptake out of the blood. Therefore, your cardiovascular system is crucial to your body's function and its response to different situations such as exercise or feeding.

WHAT IS CARDIOVASCULAR DISEASE?

Cardiovascular disease means all diseases that affect the heart and the circulation. Angina, heart attack and stroke are the three biggest diseases associated with the cardiovascular system and all have a similar underlying disease mechanism. In all three diseases there is a build-up of fatty deposits on the artery. This causes a narrowing of the artery and makes it difficult for the blood to flow through. If you consider that the artery is a hollow tube like a garden hose, if the hose is perfectly straight then the water will flow quickly through the tube but if there is a twist in it then the water will struggle to flow past the twist and the heart needs to pump harder to get the blood past the blockage. As this fatty deposit on the artery wall builds up it becomes harder to push the blood past the blockage, meaning there is a lack of oxygen-rich blood going to the heart. This causes the pain in the chest that is known as angina. If the fatty deposit breaks down under the pressure being exerted on it then a blood clot could form. This blood clot could get lodged in the artery supplying blood to the heart (causing a heart attack) or lodged in the artery supplying blood to the brain (causing a stroke).

CARDIOVASCULAR DISEASE RISK AND EXERCISE

Not all risk factors for cardiovascular disease can be changed but there is a significant number related to your lifestyle. By changing your behaviour now you can reduce your risk of developing cardiovascular disease in the long term. One of the major risk factors for cardiovascular disease is inactivity. When you are inactive your ability to deliver oxygen around the body in response to increasing skeletal muscle demand is reduced. This ability to deliver maximum oxygen during high demand (VO_2 max) is strongly related to your risk of cardiovascular disease. Taking part in exercise training will improve your body's ability to deliver oxygen and therefore lower your risk of cardiovascular disease. The heart is a muscle and just like other muscles in the body it adapts to training and becomes more efficient at pumping the blood around the body. This increased efficiency lowers blood pressure, which in turn reduces cardiovascular disease risk. Being inactive will also increase the level of circulating fats in the blood, meaning a fatty deposit is much more likely to form in the arteries. When we exercise we decrease the amount of circulating fat because the demand for energy during exercise and recovery is partially met by our fat stores. It is well known that the greater the exercise intensity the bigger the improvements in heart function.

HIGH-INTENSITY TRAINING AND THE CARDIOVASCULAR SYSTEM

High-intensity training rapidly increases VO_2 max (the ability to deliver maximum oxygen during high demand). The improvements in VO_2 max are greater with high-intensity training than with moderate-intensity training. This has been consistently found in all studies including people with coronary artery disease, congestive heart failure and metabolic syndrome. There are three potential mechanisms that have been strongly linked to improvements in VO_2 max, which regulate the enhancement in cardiovascular function. It is highly likely that it is an additive effect of all three mechanisms as all three are linked in the cell.

Contractile function

Your heart output – how much blood is pushed around the body – is controlled by the cells in the heart. The speed at which they shorten (when blood is forced out of the heart) and relax (when the heart refills with blood) controls the heart's ability to generate force. This is the contractile function of the heart. This force generation is one factor that controls the heart's output. The other factor is your heart rate. If the force generation of the heart cells is stronger then your heart rate will be lower. This balancing ensures that the same amount of blood is pumped around the body. Following high-intensity training shortening and relaxation rates of heart cells increase by 40% when the body is at rest. The effects of high-intensity training on heart contractile function is at least 100% greater than moderate intensity exercise training such as jogging. Therefore, you will have a bigger reduction in resting heart rate following high-intensity training than moderate exercise training. This is also true when you do exercise. Following high-intensity training a lower heart beat is also seen at increasing exercise intensities compared to moderate intensity training. The reason for this is the increased strength of heart cell contraction; the maximum strength of contraction is increased by up to 60% following high-intensity training. The effect on contractile function does not continue indefinitely but reaches a new stable level after about eight weeks. This occurs because either the heart cells can no longer adapt to the exercise or because the training sessions are no longer stressful enough to induce changes in the heart cells.

Calcium metabolism

Contraction of the heart muscle is a highly controlled process. The key control point of this is calcium, both outside and inside the heart cells. For the heart muscle to contract, calcium needs to enter the heart cell from the blood, which then triggers the release of more calcium from inside the heart cells. This release of calcium allows the contraction process to occur through its combination with cardiac proteins. After the contraction phase the excess calcium is removed from the heart cells and they then relax. If the heart cannot handle calcium efficiently then the heart cells cannot generate enough power and heart rate will need to increase to ensure adequate heart output. Following high-intensity training the processing of calcium through the heart cell is much more efficient, especially during the relaxation stage where free calcium is removed from the cell. There also appears to be more calcium available within the heart cells, meaning more calcium will combine with the proteins allowing a bigger contraction to occur. High-intensity training will also increase the amount of protein turnover within the heart cells promoting a better response to calcium.

Heart hypertrophy

Hypertrophy is the process where muscles get bigger. In adults this can only occur by having more proteins in the cells, resulting in the heart getting bigger. The increase in protein mass increases the heart's ability to pump blood around the body. Following high-intensity training there is an increase in heart cell protein mass that is detectable after just two weeks of training. The heart cells become about 14% bigger following high-intensity training and this is much bigger than the hypertrophy normally seen with moderate-intensity exercise, normally about 5%. Like contractile function, the heart cell growth reaches a new stable level after two months. Again, two possible explanations exist for this: either the cells have reached a maximal growth or the exercise is no longer stressing the heart to force more adaptation. The process of exercise-induced hypertrophy is controlled by an increase in the rate of conversion of messenger RNA into protein. The result of this hypertrophy is a bigger and stronger heart which can push more blood around the body. This is very different from the hypertrophy associated with disease where there is a greater increase in different gene expression and the hypertrophy impairs the heart's function.

CONCLUSION

Health is a major issue facing all of us, and it is vital that we take responsibility for our own health. The biggest chronic diseases facing society today are directly related to the lifestyle that we choose. The biggest thing we can do to improve our health is to exercise, no matter how old we are or how unfit we are. It is well known that inactivity is the biggest risk factor for developing both type 2 diabetes and heart disease. High-intensity training has consistently produced bigger effects than moderate-intensity exercise at improving outcomes associated with these diseases. Unlike moderate-intensity exercise the time required to perform the exercise is much smaller, with training sessions lasting less than 15 minutes in total, and does not need to be done as often, with health benefits shown using just two training sessions every week.

3

THE MENTAL ELEMENTS OF HIGH-INTENSITY TRAINING

You have decided to try high-intensity training. You are either going to be starting an exercise programme for the first time, incorporating this into your own established routine, or, perhaps like many people, you are starting a new programme after having stopped exercising for some time. High-intensity training is probably not like anything you have experienced before. There is no doubt that high-intensity training is physically demanding, yet unlike many challenging forms of physical activity the duration of your training sessions will be very brief. Instead of hours of running or cycling you will be training for 15 minutes at a time, at most. Instead of going out every morning or evening you will be training perhaps only three times a week to ensure your body has sufficient time to recover. High-intensity training is a unique form of exercise and comes with its own characteristic mental experiences. You need to ask yourself what you are going to have to do to make this experience a successful one. Your body might be ready for the experience, but your mental attitude is what you need to work on when it comes to working through this type of programme. If you have previously had trouble sticking with exercise it is probably the mental challenges that have stopped you.

POSITIVE MENTAL BEFITS OF EXERCISE

The previous chapters of this book have focused on the physical benefits of exercise such as increasing your performance or improving your physical health, but the psychological benefits are no less important. Engaging in an exercise programme such as high-intensity training can improve your mood, help you deal with stress and improve your self-esteem by making you feel more confident about your physical abilities.

IMPROVED MOOD

Perhaps the most widely known mental benefit of exercise is an increase in positive mood. High-intensity training, like all physical activity, causes the brain to release a number of chemicals including serotonin, norepinephrine and, most well known, endorphins. A lack of serotonin or norepinephrine in the brain is associated with depression and negative mood states. Exercise has been found to be just as effective for alleviating these moods as working with a therapist. Endorphins, which have also been called 'feel good' hormones, are thought to be responsible for what is known as the 'runner's high', a feeling of calm that accompanies strenuous physical activity, which results in a more buoyant and stable mood. Exercise also triggers the release of testosterone, which contrary to how it is portrayed as a 'male' hormone, has positive benefits for everyone, including feelings of increased confidence and personal drive.

REDUCED PAIN

The endorphins that are released during exercise can also reduce the transmission of pain impulses. They do this by attaching to receptors on the outer surfaces of brain cells and inducing a state of euphoria that blocks pain signals. This means exercise can be a great way to deal with chronic pain. The body responds this way because endorphins are produced during times of stress to allow us to run or fight despite injury and fatigue. The body interprets bouts of exercise as a stressful situation and so releases endorphins and other hormones to help us 'survive'. This means the more intensive the exercise the more powerful the endorphin response. It is also possible for your body to become accustomed to these hormones, which requires you to train at progressively more intensive levels to achieve the same effect. This means high-intensity training is an ideal training routine as it works the body at a progressively strenuous level and so induces a reciprocal level in released endorphins and other related hormones.

LOWER LEVELS OF STRESS

Starting and continuing with exercise can also act as a buffer against stress and can help protect you from some of the physical consequences of stressful events such as poor cardiovascular or immune system responses. Although exercise does not remove the source of your stress it does provide a short-term diversion from a problem and so can help reduce stress by distracting you from day-to-day issues. Regular exercise has been linked with improved sleep patterns and a reduction in levels of cortisol, sometimes called the 'stress' hormone, both of which can help improve your mood and reduce stress levels. Another way exercise can reduce stress is by increasing your feelings of control over your life which leads to improved confidence.

IMPROVED CONFIDENCE

Exercise increases your self-esteem and your feelings of self-worth. As you experience high-intensity training and master its challenges you will increase your belief in your own abilities, and as you successfully achieve increasingly more demanding sessions your self-confidence will rise. Normally, these changes come from simply sticking with the programme, but as you continue with exercise you will improve your fitness and find people responding more positively to you. Normal activities of daily living such as carrying shopping or taking the stairs will become easier and you will feel more confident about your physical ability. Knowing that you are doing something positive for yourself and that you are becoming a stronger person, both physically and mentally, will boost your overall sense of worth and self-esteem.

IMPROVED MENTAL ABILITY

Exercise can also stimulate the mind and has been shown to encourage the brain to create new brain cells known as neurons. These new neurons are generated in the hippocampus, an area of the brain which is responsible for creating and retrieving memories. Neurons form new connections between themselves, enhancing your ability to learn and to retain information. It has been shown that regular physical activity can help improve our short-term memory and cognitive abilities such as reasoning and maths skills. Exercise has also been linked with preserving existing neurons and preventing the deterioration of critical parts of the brain. Reduced flow of blood to the brain is thought to be responsible in part for a decline in our mental abilities as we age so an increase in oxygen-rich blood flow to the brain that occurs when we exercise is beneficial. This means that exercise may partially decelerate the ageing process. Exercise has also been to shown to be associated with the creation of new neurological connections in the brain to accommodate the new skills and demands of an exercise programme, which in turn can improve your reactions, your spatial awareness and your general cognitive abilities.

YOUR FIRST EXPERIENCES OF HIGH-INTENSITY TRAINING

When you first try high-intensity training you will probably have the same attitudes that many people have. A typical routine can consist of four 30-second sprints with 4-minute breaks between each, or ten to twelve 6-second sprints with 1-minute breaks. This amount of running or cycling does not sound a lot (it is only a couple of minutes of exercise in total) and the rest breaks you get sound more than long enough to recover. So what will the initial experiences actually be like?

You step up to the start line if you are running, or start getting the pedals moving if you are sprinting on a bike. You may feel apprehensive, or nervous, or perhaps even a little excited. It is going to be hard going but you know that it will be over quickly. Your heart begins to beat faster with anticipation. You look at the timer and prepare yourself. You hear the starting beep or your friend shouts 'go' and you start sprinting.

If you opted for the 30-second programme your first sprint is going to seem longer than you thought it would. Thirty seconds may not sound like a lot but when you are going flat out at maximum intensity your sense of time will distort and appear to stretch it out. You start off well pushing hard and moving fast but as the sprint goes on you feel yourself slowing down. You urge yourself to keep the pace up but your body struggles to respond. Your sprint becomes a moderate pace, then a slow pace, then a slog. Finally, the timer stops and you are finished. Your heart will be racing, your breathing quick and deep, and your legs will feel weak. You have done the first sprint and you now have four full minutes to recover. If you opted for the 6-second programme your first sprint will seem completely different and will feel easier. You start off well pushing hard, feeling yourself accelerating and getting to your top speed. Before you realise it the time is up and you have stopped. You are breathing hard, heart racing, but your legs will still feel fresh. You may feel like you are ready to go again right away and you still have a full minute to recover before you have to go again.

If you are doing the 30-second sprints you are now about halfway through your 4-minute recovery. By now you are feeling almost fully recovered and the 4-minute recovery period may seem excessively long. The first sprint was hard, but you managed, and you have recovered quickly. If you did the 6-second sprint the minute recovery will seem very short but that won't matter, as you still feel fresh. Whichever programme you are following you are now feeling positive about the next sprint and eager to get on with it and finish this session. You get yourself set to go again. You start your second sprint, running as fast as you can.

With the 30-second programme the second sprint will feel slower and harder; you reach your top speed and then begin to quickly slow down, striving to keep a steady pace. You will not go as fast as you did on your first sprint and will finish at a slower speed. Now you only have one or two sprints left to go. With the 6-second programme the second sprint will seem much the same as the first and your pace will be almost as good. However, as you finish your sprint you will be aware that you still have eight to ten of these to go.

Both programmes come with their own physical and mental challenges. For those of you doing the 30-second programme you will find the 4 minutes of recovery seem to get shorter while the sprints seem to get longer. The 30-second programme is harder than the first sprint but while these sprints will be difficult there are comparatively fewer of them. For the 6-second programme the first handful of sprints will seems very similar and you won't notice any decrease in performance but as you go on you will find that a 1-minute rest is not really all that long and you have a larger number of sprints to get through.

After you have finished either programme you are going to be physically and mentally exhausted. This was probably the most intensive training you have ever done.

Looking down at your watch you will be amazed that so little time has past. Only 10 to 15 minutes have gone by but you feel like you have been training a lot longer. How are you feeling? Well, you are probably thinking that you cannot physically run any more and even the idea of walking back to the changing room seems like a lot of effort. Your legs will be shaky and you may be feeling a little nauseous especially if you have eaten anything before the session began. For some minutes after finishing, your heart will continue to race and you will be breathing hard. You are probably sitting down.

You are pleased that you did not stop and that you are finished but you are probably thinking that perhaps once was enough and you are not convinced you will be carrying on with this training. Yet over the next few hours something will happen to change that attitude completely. You will become more and more satisfied with the fact that you completed all of your sprints and genuinely pleased with what you have accomplished. Perhaps only a few hours after completing the training you will already be starting to look forward to the next session. You will be thinking that it did not really feel that bad and that it was over really quickly. After a full day of rest you will be keen for your next session. Once again you may feel a certain amount of apprehension but it will be tinged with more excitement. You will be eager to see if you can do better than last time. Can you go faster or further? As you progress from session to session you will observe improvements in your performance such as running faster and recovering more quickly as you master your own fitness. Although the sprints will be hard, and they will often be physically exhausting, they will be rewarding. During each training session everything will be focused on pushing hard, your life stresses will become distant and forgotten, to be replaced with a flood of endorphins.

COPING WITH THE CHALLENGES OF HIGH-INTENSITY TRAINING

High-intensity training is a rewarding but physically demanding exercise programme. Even if you have previously been involved in exercise and consider yourself fit, high-intensity training is unlike any other type of physical activity you are likely to have been involved in. Weariness, fatigue and soreness are all typical during high-intensity training but to achieve our goals we have to push our limitations, and the greatest satisfaction comes from overcoming our own personal boundaries and accomplishing more than we thought we could. High-intensity training is made up of repeated bursts of strenuous activity followed by inactivity as you rest. It is a distinctive type of training that you will need to be mentally prepared for. So, how do you cope with it?

THE PROBLEMS WITH JUST 'DOING YOUR BEST'

The purpose of high-intensity training is to sprint for a set time period, for example, 30 seconds or 6 seconds. This means running or cycling at your maximum pace. Effectively, you are being asked to 'do your best', to push yourself as hard as you can. In each sprint you really have no fixed goal to achieve but instead you are trying to continue at maximum for the full duration – you have no set distance to cover, no top speed or peak cycling

RPM to achieve. This is the way it should be as you should always be trying to work as hard as you possibly can. You may be better or faster on some days than others but you should always be trying your hardest. However, it is not as simple as that. When people are asked to work as hard as they can during exercise they often set spontaneous goals such as covering a certain distance or reaching a certain point during a sprint. The basic assumption of goals is that your performance is regulated directly by the targets you set and your achievement of them. Hence, upon reaching a goal many people will stop, or reduce their effort, which in turn limits the effectiveness and benefits of the high-intensity training.

People undertaking any form of physical activity will often spontaneously set goals, particularly when given some form of performance feedback by which to judge their achievement. In our own research using hill-sprinting outside we found that many people would privately pick a point, a cone or a tree, that they wanted to reach as a minimum distance during their sprint. This seemed to limit their performance and most of those involved did not see any improvement in the distance they were covering during their sprints despite a large increase in their fitness levels over two weeks of training. We think this was because upon reaching that minimum distance they stopped trying so hard. Spontaneous goals can also have other negative influences on you. If you are looking at a stopwatch or clock or you have a well-meaning friend shouting out how long you have to go, then you have access to a way to evaluate your own performance during the sprint. There is nothing worse than hearing you still have half the sprint to go when you are already feeling the strain and have not covered as far as you thought you would. This can be very disheartening and can again result in reduced effort and poorer results. If you are going to seriously try high-intensity training you need to find ways to ensure you give your maximum effort each time, regardless of how good or bad that may be.

DISSOCIATION AND ASSOCIATION

The most commonly employed strategy in exercise is known as *dissociation*. Dissociation is about distracting yourself from what is going on. This means mentally disconnecting from the weariness or discomfort and ignoring bodily sensations that may hold you back. There are a number of possible dissociative strategies that can be used. The most obvious example in exercise is one almost everyone uses and that is listening to music. Music can both distract us and motivate us and should be picked carefully. A classic orchestral piece is not likely to make you sprint any faster and a thumping rock song is not likely to help you rest and relax between sprints. Some people will distract themselves by chatting to friends or will focus on the end result, thinking about how good they will feel when they finish the training session, the nice meal they will cook when they get home or how happy they will be when they get fitter.

A less commonly employed strategy is *association*. This is where you focus on what you are doing and concentrate on doing as well as you can. This means monitoring your body and being very much in the moment. Associative strategies include paying attention to the parts of the body under most exertion, such as your legs, focusing on your technique, trying to pedal or run as fast you can, or concentrating on maintaining a steady rhythm and pace as you begin to tire. Focusing on your body's sensations can help you to reframe or reinterpret the signals of your body, seeing them not as weariness or strain, but as positive signals that you are really doing your best and getting the most out of each training session. It also means you can prevent yourself from pushing your limits too far and overdoing it, changing your pace and reacting to any warning signals from your body.

Dissociation and distracting yourself has been linked to lower feelings of fatigue in exercise, suggesting that these strategies can increase our ability to keep going through physical activity. However, this has only been seen in relatively low-intensity endurance situations such as long runs. Dissociation does not allow an individual to work at a higher intensity or to overcome high levels of fatigue and pain. Distractions then are not good when trying to work at a high intensity. Perhaps the worst distraction is focusing on how much time is left during a sprint; this is often disheartening and can be counter-productive and lead to less effort towards the end of each sprint. Dissociation is a useful tool for reducing weariness and discomfort, however, when the intensity of effort is very high, it has been shown to be less effective. Associative strategies allow individuals to perform at a higher level of intensity meaning faster sprints and increased effort. Does this mean that when doing high-intensity training you should avoid dissociation and exclusively use association? The answer is no; both have their place.

During the actual sprints themselves, where the going is particularly tough, associative strategies lead to increased performance as individuals can gauge their body's limitations and reinterpret the unavoidable levels of discomfort that come from exercising at a high level. Conversely, during rest periods dissociation is a useful method for reducing weariness and discomfort, helping maintain motivation by distracting you from the repeated demanding bouts of activity. Practically, this means you need to set up your training sessions to allow for both strategies. During the sprint you need to minimise distractions. The easiest way to do this is to have an automatic timer that beeps at the end of the sprint duration or have a friend hold a stopwatch and to shout out when you need to stop. Minimise distractions and focus on pumping those legs and going as fast as you can during each sprint. Conversely, during the rest period you want to be distracted. Your legs are likely to hurt and you do not want to think about having to do it again. Listen to music or chat with friends. However, make sure your friends know what kind of support you need. Our own group is very competitive and the chat can often be quite sharp and verge on mocking each other's performance. This works for some while others need more encouragement and support.

Everyone needs different mental strategies to get them through exercise. Think about what you do and which of the two categories described fits best. Have you been using the right strategies and do you need to change anything? A well-motivated exerciser will use both, changing from one to the other where needed. Use association to maximise your efforts and use dissociation to distract you and to stave off the monotony of sustained training.

MAINTAINING MOTIVATION

Getting motivated to start a new exercise programme like high-intensity training is easy when you are planning it out. It is easy to get excited about the training and to convince yourself that this is exactly what you need to get your fitness and your health back on track. It is not so easy when the alarm clock goes off and you actually have to get out of bed and go and do it. It can be even harder after you have done your first high-intensity training and realised that although economical in terms of time it requires a lot of physical and mental effort from you. All the reasons you had for starting the exercise programme can start to seem less important and other aspects of your life suddenly seem much more important than going out and training. You may be wondering why some people stick with exercise and others struggle to maintain a healthy routine. A lack of motivation may be the single greatest barrier between you and all the benefits high-intensity training can provide. If so, you need to work out exactly what it is that will keep you training and maintain your interest.

OVERCOMING BARRIERS

Throughout your training programme you will be confronted with distractions and potential excuses to do less or even to give up. Perhaps you have a busy time at work or maybe you need to spend more time with your family. High-intensity training naturally overcomes two of the biggest barriers to exercise – time and money – as it is so quick to do and can be done with little or no equipment. However, you must still prepare yourself to

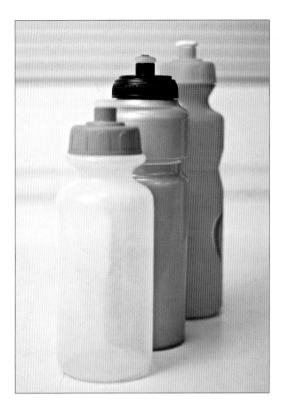

Hydration is important but make sure you
do not drink too much before your workout.

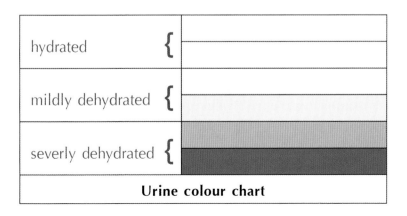

hydrated {	
mildly dehydrated {	
severly dehydrated {	
Urine colour chart	

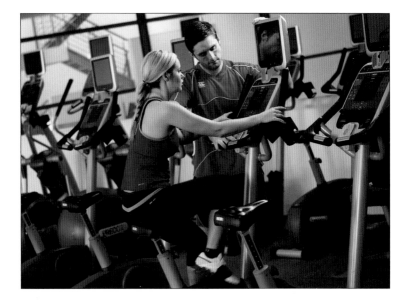

When using a gym bike, you might find it easier to have a partner control the intensity whilst you concentrate on going as fast as you can.

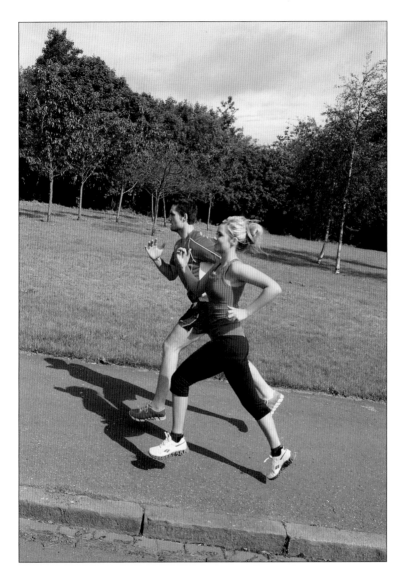

You might find it easier to maintain your
motivation if you train with a partner.

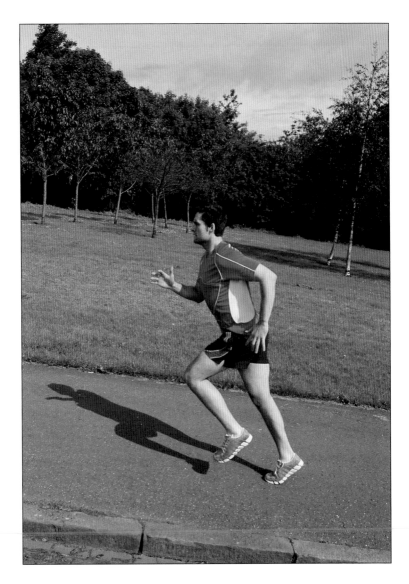

Make sure you give maximum effort in every sprint.

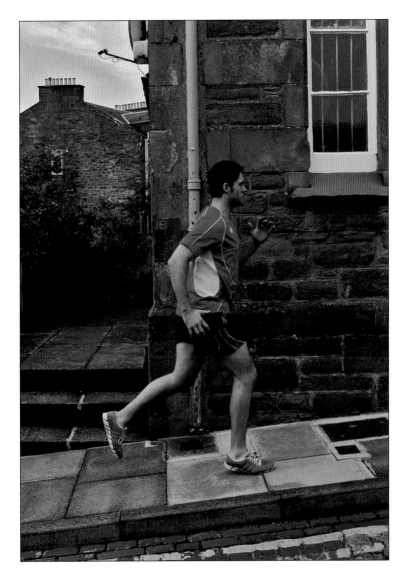

You do not need a gym for this workout, all you need is a hill and you could even do it in your own street.

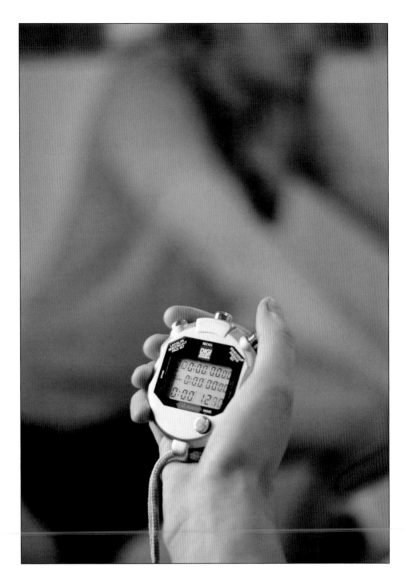

If you are using a stopwatch to time your sprints,
it is easier if you have a partner let you know
when to start and finish.

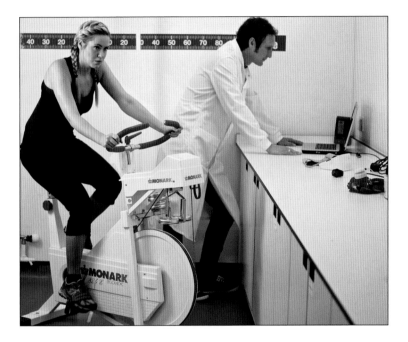

The high intensity workout is based on research being carried out in research institutes around the world.

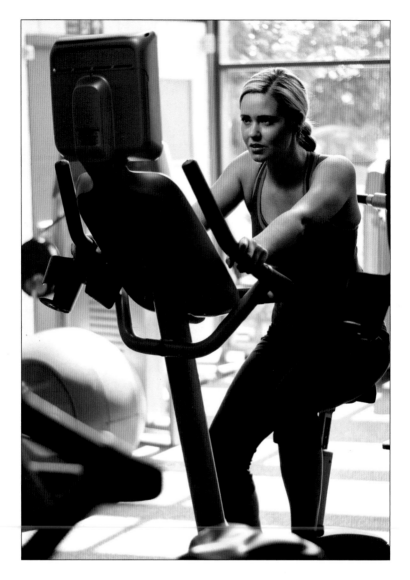

If you are already a member of a gym, why
not include the high intensity workout
as part of your training routine.

overcome barriers. When the going gets tough we often look for excuses not to do it. Sit down and write a list of all of the potential excuses you like to use and write down a solution to each excuse. Busy time at work? Perhaps you can do your training over your lunch break? After all, it only takes 10 to 15 minutes. Can't make it to the gym? Why not try doing your sprints on the hill behind your house? You should think about each excuse and have a plan to overcome it.

SOCIAL SUPPORT

Having someone to push you on is the perfect way to maintain a good exercise programme. On the days you cannot be bothered they will push you to train and you can do the same for them on their less motivated days. Having a friend along is also ideal as they can monitor the time and leave you to focus on running or cycling as fast as you can. Friends can also help you overcome some potential barriers. If you have young children, they can watch them while you do your training and vice versa. If you pick the right programme they can even run while you rest, helping maintain each other's motivation and making the workout even more time effective. So, call a friend and convince them to give high-intensity training a try with you.

FLEXIBILITY

You also need to realise that your exercise performance is going to fluctuate. Some days you will be able to push harder than others and some days you will feel like you cannot put much effort in at all. If you are completely exhausted you do not always have to complete your full programme. Listen to your body. This is fine as long as you are trying your hardest and you should not allow yourself to be put off by it. Also, some of those barriers previously discussed can become real reasons and not excuses for avoiding exercise. Say you scheduled a training session for your lunch break but then your boss tells you an important deadline has been moved forward. You do not need to stick pedantically to your schedule. Can you do the session after work? Can you miss the cycling session at the gym and instead do a sprinting session on a hill near where you live? For many people it is all or nothing and they will end up skipping a training session rather than coming up with an alternative. You need to be willing to be flexible and to change your routine. Think again about the barriers you may face and see if you can come up with a backup plan.

MONITORING AND PROGRESSION

You will maintain your motivation longer if you can see the benefits of your training programme. One good approach is to keep an exercise log. Write down how often you exercise, any problems you had, and record how well you did (how far did you go, how fast were your sprints). This will help you to chart your progress and see how well you are doing. It can also help to identify reasons why you have progressed more in some weeks than others. Another idea is to take a picture of yourself each month in your training clothes. This gives you a visual record of body changes and progress to go into your log. Your body will change when you do high-intensity training but sometimes the changes happen slowly and you do not notice them. A picture log can help you see what is happening and how you are improving. As you progress you can also use your log to update your training routine. This can add excitement and challenge to your workout especially if training with friends and a little bit of friendly competition can really help motivation. Monitoring your routine and keeping it updated will also help to prevent you reaching a plateau and wasting your time without seeing any improvements.

SETTING APPROPRIATE GOALS FOR YOUR TRAINING

Ask yourself why are you exercising. You need to be doing this for yourself. Perhaps you are trying to lose weight for an upcoming event like a wedding, or perhaps you are worried about your health, or maybe you just want a new challenge. Think about how these reasons motivate you and how they may change over time. If your reason for exercising is based upon anyone other than yourself you need to re-evaluate what you are doing. Trying to lose weight because you are worried about what your friends or partner think is never going to sustain your motivation through even the easiest of exercise programme and especially not one based on high-intensity training. Establish exactly what you are trying to achieve and what you are going to do to accomplish it. Write down these goals and place them somewhere where you will see them every day, on your desk at work or by the mirror in your bedroom. You need to do this to remind yourself of your commitment to exercise and the goals you have set yourself.

THINK TODAY, NOT TOMORROW

Effective goals are about your development rather than outcomes. Focusing on your own improvement will see your confidence increase along with your fitness and health. Each training session takes you another small step towards your intermediate or overall goals. Focus on small steps such as 'I will do three training sessions this week' rather than big steps such as 'I will lose 10kg'. Remember that attaining your ideal fitness level is a process not a single event.

MAKE IT CHALLENGING, BUT MAKE IT ACHIEVABLE

Accomplishing goals raises your confidence and increases your motivation, but for them to work you have to succeed. If you set very hard goals like 'I will lose 5kg a week' you are setting yourself up to fail which will sap your motivation. However, if you set easy goals and achieve your goals effortlessly your motivation is also unlikely to increase. You want to succeed but you want to feel like you have had to work for it. Set challenging goals – not unrealistic or undemanding ones.

BE SPECIFIC

Goals that are too general are not going to help you get fit and healthy. Something like 'I want to be fitter' is too broad and is unlikely to be realised. A goal must be measurable so you know when you have achieved it. A specific goal should be more like 'I will be able to complete four sprints by week 5', or 'I will lose 1kg a week'. You need to have clear goals that can be assessed.

BE POSITIVE

Goals need to be about what you will do and they need to be positive. Try to avoid goals like 'I will try not to skip training sessions' and instead say 'I will go to all of my training sessions'. You want to focus your attention on doing it right and not on potential mistakes or barriers. Goals are like prophecies; whatever you draw attention to is more likely to happen. Try to word your goals positively to maximise their ability to motivate you. Write them down and stick to them.

CONCLUSION

Making the decision to begin high-intensity training is the first step. Fitness and health is often the last thing on our daily agenda but by reading this you are taking a positive step in your life and physical training. Although you will face many mental and physical challenges while doing this training, if you have prepared properly and thought carefully about your motivations and potential barriers then there is no reason for you not to succeed. High-intensity training offers many potential benefits and as you progress you will find more energy and enthusiasm, and will develop a more positive mental attitude in your life.

4

PRACTICAL ASPECTS OF HIGH-INTENSITY TRAINING

You now understand the science behind high-intensity training and recognise that it is not the latest fad but a highly efficient way to improve your general fitness levels and gain important health improvements. This chapter will provide you with practical considerations that you may not have thought about and some simple protocols to start you on the road to starting a successful high-intensity training programme. Like all training regimes you get out of it exactly what you put in. If you do not carry out the sprints as an all-out effort then the usefulness of the training will be lost and at the end of the day you will only be deceiving yourself.

EATING AND DRINKING BEFORE, DURING AND AFTER YOUR HIGH-INTENSITY WORKOUT

Due to the nature of high-intensity exercise it is important that you do not perform the training session after having eaten. Eating a short time before any exercise can make you sluggish, because of the energy requirements associated with digesting food. For example, to digest a meal containing 400 calories requires approximately 33% more blood flow and fuel to the gut to allow the intestinal tract to extract the nutrients. This means that there is less blood flow and fuel available to the skeletal muscles performing the exercise, in turn meaning that your performance will be impaired. This may be to such an extent that you are not able to complete the full high-intensity workout. The nutritional committee of the International Olympic Committee (IOC) recommends that for elite-level athletes their last intake of food should consist mainly of carbohydrates and occur at least four hours before performing exercise, which is sufficient time to allow the fuel to be transported into the blood stream. This is also good advice for the non-elite athlete or the person just looking to become more active. For a high-intensity workout it is really important that digestion is complete.

Water intake before exercise is critical to allow you to perform to your maximum. Mild dehydration has been shown to reduce performance by as much as 10% and the more dehydrated you are the worse your performance will be. The easiest way to determine your hydration level is to look at the colour of your urine at least three hours before your planned session. If you are hydrated your urine should be a light straw-yellow colour, getting darker the more dehydrated you are. Compare your urine colour to the colour chart shown in the plate section. The IOC nutritional committee recommends that 500ml of water should be consumed two hours before exercise to ensure optimal hydration before exercise. This allows time for the water to be extracted from the gut (a process which takes approximately one hour depending on the volume of water taken). Taking in water any closer to exercise will mean that the gut is still working to extract it and you will not be hydrated before you start exercising. For a high-intensity workout you should try to avoid taking in water three hours before exercise. This is to ensure that the gut is completely free of excessive fluid before you start the session. If you have excessive fluid in your stomach before you start a high-intensity workout then you will feel uncomfortable and may possibly even vomit during the session.

During the high-intensity workout you will not become dehydrated, your internal body temperature will hardly be raised and you will not sweat very much at all (dependent on the temperature of the room or the temperature outside). There is no need to drink fluids between the sprints, however, you may experience a dry mouth towards the later sprints in the workout. This is not due to dehydration but because you will breath through your mouth during the sprints rather than through your nose. If this happens and you can't wait until the end of the workout then you can have a very small sip of water between the sprints, but try not to drink too much water.

After the high-intensity workout your legs should feel like they are empty and you need to start refuelling your skeletal muscles to allow a fast recovery from the workout. The key to this recovery is to provide both carbohydrate and protein after the workout. The provision of carbohydrate will begin the process of replacing the skeletal muscle glycogen that has been used. Immediately after the workout skeletal muscle is exceptionally sensitive to glucose and early intake of carbohydrate will lead to a rapid recovery of the skeletal muscles' glycogen stores. The provision of protein after the workout will stimulate protein synthesis in the skeletal muscles which will lead to improvements in the functionality of the skeletal muscle. The provision of carbohydrate and protein could be done by having a balanced lunch/dinner following the workout or by drinking a protein and carbohydrate supplement. These supplements have a strong scientific rationale but are unnecessary if you are going to eat a meal after the session. A cheaper alternative, which has been shown to be the most effective exercise recovery drink, is milk.

HOW LONG SHOULD EACH SPRINT BE AND HOW MANY SHOULD BE IN A WORKOUT?

We have seen in previous chapters that performance and health benefits can be accrued with either short duration sprints of 6 to 10 seconds in duration or with longer duration sprints lasting 30 seconds. Other studies have used longer duration sprint protocols but there appears to be no added benefit; therefore I would not recommend doing any sprint sessions where the sprint lasts for longer than 30 seconds. Doing sprints for longer than 30 seconds would be unpleasant, as well. The choice between short and long-duration sprints is for you to make but when starting out on a high-intensity training scheme for the first time, I would advise you to use one of the shorter sprint protocols to allow your body to get used to the demands of the exercise. This is true for people wanting to become active or for people who are already active and seeking to improve their performance. We still cannot say which protocol produces the biggest improvements in either fitness or health. As research continues into high-intensity training we will get a much better idea about what protocols are the most effective.

Like all exercise training programmes, you should use a progressive approach where you increase the number of sprints until you are performing ten short-duration sprints or four to six longer-duration sprints. With the 6-second sprint protocol a typical progressive schedule would start with six sprints and build up to ten sprints over four weeks. With the 30-second sprint protocol a typical progressive schedule would start with two sprints and build up to four sprints over four weeks. If you increase the number of sprints above this then the amount of time required for the workout increases and the time efficiency of the high-intensity workout disappears. The purpose of any exercise training is to make the body do work that it is not used to doing, that is, stressing the body, so that the body adapts to the stress placed on it and improvements in fitness will occur. Likewise, this stressing of the body and adaptation will also be responsible for the health improvements that are seen with exercise. However, training is only beneficial if it is forcing the body, especially skeletal muscle, to adapt and once you have been training for a while you reach a level of performance and fitness which is difficult to increase any further. If the stress of training is too low then no adaptation will occur and if it is too great then injury is a real possibility. Being aware of this at the beginning your training programme will ensure the desired adaptations occur rapidly and without injury.

HOW MUCH TIME SHOULD I LEAVE FOR RECOVERY BETWEEN EACH SPRINT IN A TRAINING SESSION?

The amount of time that you leave between each sprint depends on what length of sprint you are using for your training session. For a 6-second sprint you would normally leave 1 minute for recovery, but for a 30-second sprint you should leave a minimum of 4 minutes' recovery. Therefore, when you are training you need to alter your recovery period to reflect the duration of the sprints you are using in the workout. The recovery period between each sprint is exceptionally important as it allows the skeletal muscles' 'fast-use fuel systems' (adenosine triphosphate stores and phosphocreatine stores) to recover before doing the next sprint to ensure you can perform optimally in each sprint in the training session. If you do not allow enough recovery time between the sprints then you will not be able to produce similar intensities in each sprint during the training session. You can see on page 76 that the amount of power you can produce in the second sprint is much less when the recovery period is not long enough. As we saw in chapter 1, skeletal muscle has different sources that it will utilise to maintain its energy source, adenosine triphosphate, during exercise. One of the major sources of adenosine triphosphate production during a sprint is the phosphocreatine system. This system is exceptionally important for generating the initial power produced by the skeletal muscle. The longer your sprint lasts, the more phosphocreatine you use. This is demonstrated on page 76 where you can see the use of phosphocreatine during the sprint and the time taken to recover. We use most of the phosphocreatine in the muscle within the first 15 seconds

THE HIGH INTENSITY WORKOUT

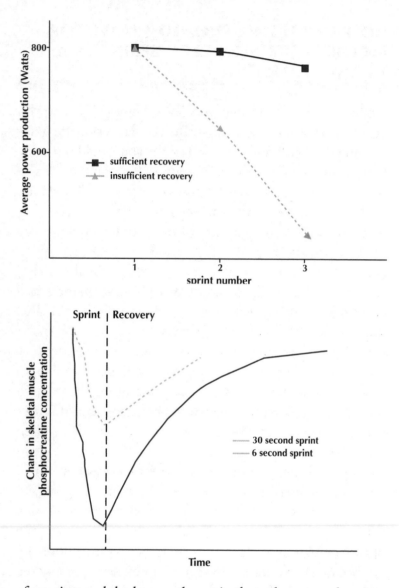

of a sprint, and the longer the sprint lasts the more glycogen is used. It takes approximately 15 to 20 minutes to fully recover phosphocreatine but approximately 90% is recovered in 4 minutes. The other main fuel source for this type of exercise, glycogen, will not start to recover until you begin to eat carbohydrates following the training session.

HOW SHOULD I RECOVER BETWEEN EACH SPRINT?

There are two things you can do when you finish your first sprint. You can either perform low-intensity exercise (known as active recovery) or you can remain stationary (known as passive recovery). There is a considerable use of both adenosine triphosphate and phosphocreatine during a high-intensity sprint. The priorities for skeletal muscle during recovery are to replenish the adenosine triphosphate and phosphocreatine stores. The replenishment of these stores prepares the skeletal muscle for any subsequent increase in use; during a high-intensity workout this will be the next sprint. It has long been established that a major factor for control of phosphocreatine replenishment is the speed at which blood is delivered to the skeletal muscles used during the exercise. In experiments where the blood flow to the legs is restricted, the replenishment of phosphocreatine does not happen. The important component of blood for phosphocreatine replenishment is oxygen. Delivering adequate oxygen to the recovering skeletal muscle promotes the production of an excess of adenosine triphosphate from glucose and fats which can be used to turn creatine back to phosphocreatine. As well as delivering oxygen the blood also takes away so-called waste products that normalise the environment within the muscle cells and improve the processing of fuel during subsequent bouts of exercise.

One way to promote increased blood flow to the

recovering skeletal muscles is to perform low-intensity exercise using the previously exercised muscles, that is, to do an active recovery. But is this any better than a passive recovery? The evidence suggests that when you are performing repeated bouts of high-intensity exercise lasting for 30 seconds or less, an active recovery is more beneficial than a passive recovery. Using an active recovery protocol will keep the heart rate higher than a passive recovery protocol ensuring increased delivery of oxygen to the skeletal muscles and improved normalisation of the muscle cell environment. It has been shown that an active recovery will increase phosphocreatine replenishment and improve the use of glycogen during the subsequent sprint, which allows you to generate more power during the sprints which will give a bigger training adaptation.

In practical terms this means that you should keep moving after each sprint. The type of sprints you are doing will determine the type of recovery. If you are using a bike then you need to pedal at a low speed against a very low resistance, if you are performing running sprints then a slow walk back to the start is an adequate way to recover. Be sure to keep moving if you get back to the start line before your recovery time is over.

HOW MANY TIMES A WEEK SHOULD I PERFORM A HIGH-INTENSITY WORKOUT?

Doing too much training every week will not allow the body enough time to recover between workouts and will have a detrimental effect on your performance. This is known as overtraining. Adaptation of the body to the workout starts immediately after you have finished the session and, depending on the intensity of the session, can take 48 hours to complete. If you do not allow sufficient recovery between workouts then you will not get the full adaptation and your performance will steadily get worse. There are some tell-tale signs to look out for as warnings of overtraining.

- poor sleep pattern
- general aches and pains in the skeletal muscles or joints
- a general feeling of tiredness
- a lack of motivation and energy
- an increased susceptibility to illnesses such as cold
- a decrease in performance

If you experience any of these warning signs you need to stop exercising and have a few days of rest to recover.

Due to the nature of the high-intensity workout – an all-out, maximal-effort training session – you can run the risk of overtraining if you do not allow sufficient recovery time between each workout. From studies it is clear that a minimum of 24 hours should be left between each high-intensity workout. Failure to leave this amount of recovery will result in much smaller gains in skeletal muscle performance from the same amount of training. Therefore, with a high-intensity workout you are looking for no more than three training sessions per week with at least 24 hours between each session to allow your body the time that is needed to adapt to the stress of the exercise. To fit the amount of exercise that you wish to do in a week means that you need to plan your week in advance, fitting in sessions as best you can around your work/family commitments, then rearrange accordingly to afford as much recovery time as possible between your sessions. You may even want to get your family involved in timing your sprint bouts and recovery times.

HOW CAN I DO HIGH-INTENSITY TRAINING?

Most of the research that has been carried out on high-intensity training has used electronically braked static bikes that are normally found in sports science laboratories and not available to the general population. These bikes can finely control the intensity of the exercise but they are not necessary to produce equally good improvement in fitness and health. There are protocols that have been used that do not require these bikes.

RUNNING

The easiest way to do a high-intensity workout is to sprint uphill. Uphill sprinting has been shown to be just as effective at improving fitness as the traditional 30-second static bike sprint protocol. When you perform uphill sprints the intensity of the exercise is controlled by the slope of the hill. The steeper the slope of a hill, the harder you will need to work to drive your body up it. Also, the more you weigh the harder the session will be. This is because the work that you do is directly related to the mass that you are trying to move (force = mass x acceleration). Some practical workouts are given later in this chapter. You can control your session by either running between two fixed points such as trees or by using a stopwatch to give a specific time that you will sprint for. If you are sprinting between two fixed points then you need to know how long this has taken you to allow yourself sufficient recovery time. If you are using a stopwatch it is better if you have a countdown facility to stop you from looking at the watch during the sprint.

If you do not have access to any suitable hills then you can still perform a high-intensity running workout using either a weighted vest or a weighted rucksack to increase the intensity of the exercise. A weighted vest is more comfortable to run with but can cost a lot of money. A well-fitted walking rucksack with added weights secured around your middle will provide a much cheaper way to increase the intensity. If you do not own weights then you could add bags of sugar or salt to the rucksack to increase the intensity.

GYM BIKE

The typical static bike found in a gym uses air resistance to control the intensity. This means that unless the manufacturer develops a high-intensity protocol then it is quite difficult to control the resistance. If you are going to use a gym bike then it is beneficial to have a training partner. It is not impossible to do it on your own but it is much simpler if you have someone to help. Due to how these bikes work it is difficult to cycle at a high enough intensity (anything above 110RPM) and try and hold down the resistance switch to increase the intensity. With practice it gets easier. The other disadvantage of using a gym bike is that there is a limited resistance to which you can cycle against which will limit its usefulness in the long term as your body adapts to the training.

SWIMMING

A 25m all-out-effort swim will be likely to have similar adaptations to the traditional cycle protocols. This is because the skeletal muscles in the body have to work against the resistance of the water to propel you forward. The faster you try to move through the water, the harder the body will have to work, placing more stress on the body and getting a bigger adaptation. However, you cannot change the intensity of the swim, which means the only way you can increase the intensity is to increase the number of sprints you do in a session. This will eventually lead to you losing the time efficiency of this type of exercise.

WHEN SHOULD I CHANGE MY TRAINING SESSIONS?

Like all training schedules, if you do not change the training programme you will stop improving and move into a maintenance phase where you keep the new level of fitness that you have but you will not get any better. At some point you should look to change what you are doing, but when should you do this? With high-intensity training you will continue to see improvements for four to six weeks following the same training schedule. After this point you should seek to gradually increase the intensity of your workout. There is no definite point at which you should increase the intensity of your training, but if you listen to your body you will know when that point is. If you finish your high-intensity workout and you have found the session relatively easy, for example, your breathing recovers much quicker than previously or your legs do not feel tired, then that is when you should increase the intensity of the workout by changing from beginners' protocols to intermediate and so on.

HIGH-INTENSITY TRAINING PROGRAMMES

This section will give you some simple high-intensity programmes for you to try out. These protocols are meant to be a starting point to your high-intensity workouts. All sprints in these protocols should be performed as an all out effort for the full duration of the sprint. If you are doing the longer duration sprints you should fully expect to slow down as the sprint continues (normally after about 8 seconds). Once you become comfortable with the training schedules then you can adjust the intensity as you feel. Do not be afraid to pick and choose what you do to fit in with the amount of time that you have. If you only have 10 minutes then you may want to do fewer sprints but against a greater intensity to ensure the stress placed on the body is big enough to make the body adapt and continue to ensure improvements in fitness and health outcomes. There is no need for a warm-up before starting these sessions, but if you want to do so, keep it short: cycle warm-up – 2-minute cycle against as little resistance as possible; run warm-up – 2-minute walk or slow run; swim warm-up – 2 lengths of the pool at a slow pace.

UPHILL SPRINTING

There are two ways to control the sprints that are performed; either use a set distance (which is easier on your own) or use a set time. Both are given in the following protocols. Remember the slope of the hill is what controls the intensity, so start on a relatively shallow slope (approximately 5% gradient).

Short duration (beginner)

WEEK 1&2	TIME (SEC)	DISTANCE (M)
sprint	6	50
rest	60	walk to start
sprint	6	50
rest	60	walk to start
sprint	6	50
rest	60	walk to start
sprint	6	50
rest	60	walk to start
sprint	6	50

WEEK 3	TIME (SEC)	DISTANCE (M)
sprint	6	50
rest	60	walk to start
sprint	6	50
rest	60	walk to start
sprint	6	50

rest	60	walk to start
sprint	6	50
rest	60	walk to start
sprint	6	50
rest	60	walk to start
sprint	6	50
rest	60	walk to start
sprint	6	50
rest	60	walk to start
sprint	6	50
rest	60	walk to start
sprint	6	50
rest	60	walk to start
sprint	6	50

Long duration (beginner)

WEEK 1&2	TIME (SEC)	DISTANCE (M)
sprint	30	150
rest	240	walk to start
sprint	30	150
rest	240	walk to start
sprint	30	150

THE HIGH INTENSITY WORKOUT

WEEK 3	TIME (SEC)	DISTANCE (M) (ON BIKE AT 110RPM)
sprint	30	150
rest	240	walk to start
sprint	30	150
rest	240	walk to start
sprint	30	150
rest	240	walk to start
sprint	30	150

Once you become comfortable with these protocols on a shallow hill it is time to increase the intensity. The easiest way to do this is to find a steeper hill and repeat the four or ten sprint sessions outlined above. If this option is not available then you need to add weight as explained above. When you increase the intensity you should seek to work at this new intensity for at least four weeks before changing the training sessions.

GYM BIKE

These protocols are designed for gym bikes where the top resistance level is 20. Before increasing the resistance it is really important that you bring your cycling speed up to at least 110RPM.

Short duration (beginner)

WEEK 1	TIME (SEC)	RESISTANCE LEVEL
sprint	6	15
rest	60	1
sprint	6	15
rest	60	1
sprint	6	15
rest	60	1
sprint	6	15
rest	60	1
sprint	6	15

WEEK 2	TIME (SEC)	RESISTANCE LEVEL
sprint	6	15
rest	60	1
sprint	6	15
rest	60	1
sprint	6	15
rest	60	1
sprint	6	15
rest	60	1
sprint	6	15
rest	60	1
sprint	6	15
rest	60	1

THE HIGH INTENSITY WORKOUT

sprint	6	15
rest	60	1
sprint	6	15
rest	60	1
sprint	6	15
rest	60	1
sprint	6	15

Long duration (beginner)

WEEK 1	TIME (SEC)	RESISTANCE LEVEL
sprint	30	15
rest	240	1
sprint	30	15
rest	240	1
sprint	30	15

WEEK 2	TIME (SEC)	RESISTANCE LEVEL
sprint	30	15
rest	240	1
sprint	30	15
rest	240	1
sprint	30	15
rest	240	1
sprint	30	15

Once you feel comfortable with these sprints against 6% of your body weight then it is time to change to a more challenging sprint workout.

Short duration (intermediate)

ALL WEEKS	TIME (SEC)	RESISTANCE LEVEL
sprint	6	17
rest	60	3
sprint	6	17
rest	60	3
sprint	6	17
rest	60	3
sprint	6	17
rest	60	3
sprint	6	17
rest	60	3
sprint	6	17
rest	60	3
sprint	6	17
rest	60	3
sprint	6	17
rest	60	3
sprint	6	17
rest	60	3
sprint	6	17

Long duration (intermediate)

ALL WEEKS	TIME (SEC)	RESISTANCE LEVEL
sprint	30	17
rest	240	3
sprint	30	17
rest	240	3
sprint	30	17
rest	240	3
sprint	30	17

You would look to follow this protocol for at least four weeks. After that, the best way to alter the protocol is to add more resistance onto each sprint, that is, change the resistance from 17 to 18 and continue with the new protocol for at least another four weeks before considering changing the intensity again. You will soon run out of resistance levels on the gym bike. You could alter the protocol by adding in extra sprints or by changing the recovery period to give slightly less rest (45 seconds on a 6-second sprint or 210 seconds on a 30-second sprint).

SWIMMING

This swimming protocol is based on research and is based on a 25m-length pool.

Beginner

WEEK 1&2	TIME (SEC)	DISTANCE (M)
sprint	20	25
rest	180	
sprint	20	25
rest	180	
sprint	20	25
rest	180	
sprint	20	25
rest	180	
sprint	20	25

Once you become comfortable with these protocols then it is time to increase the intensity. You should look to bring the number of sprints up to eight until this feels comfortable. After this, you should look to reduce the recovery time down to 120 seconds between each sprint.

TRADITIONAL WEIGHTED CRADLE STATIC BIKE

If you are lucky enough to have access to these types of static bike, for example, Monark, Watt or Lode, these are the traditional high-intensity protocols. You need to programme the bikes to add the resistance to the bike once you are pedalling at 110RPM.

Short duration (beginner)

WEEK 1	TIME (SEC)	RESISTANCE (ON BIKE AT 110RPM)
sprint	6	6% body weight
rest	60	0% body weight
sprint	6	6% body weight
rest	60	0% body weight
sprint	6	6% body weight
rest	60	0% body weight
sprint	6	6% body weight
rest	60	0% body weight
sprint	6	6% body weight

WEEK 2	TIME (SEC)	RESISTANCE (ON BIKE AT 110RPM)
sprint	6	6% body weight
rest	60	0% body weight
sprint	6	6% body weight
rest	60	0% body weight
sprint	6	6% body weight
rest	60	0% body weight
sprint	6	6% body weight
rest	60	0% body weight

sprint	6	6% body weight
rest	60	0% body weight
sprint	6	6% body weight
rest	60	0% body weight
sprint	6	6% body weight
rest	60	0% body weight
sprint	6	6% body weight
rest	60	0% body weight
sprint	6	6% body weight
rest	60	0% body weight
sprint	6	6% body weight

Long duration (beginner)

WEEK 1	TIME (SEC)	RESISTANCE (ON BIKE AT 110RPM)
sprint	30	6% body weight
rest	240	0% body weight
sprint	30	6% body weight
rest	240	0% body weight
sprint	30	6% body weight

WEEK 2	TIME (SEC)	RESISTANCE (ON BIKE AT 110RPM)
sprint	30	6% body weight
rest	240	0% body weight
sprint	30	6% body weight

THE HIGH INTENSITY WORKOUT

rest	240	0% body weight
sprint	30	6% body weight
rest	240	0% body weight
sprint	30	6% body weight

Once you feel comfortable with these sprints against 6% of your body weight then it is time to change to a more challenging sprint workout.

Short duration (intermediate)

ALL WEEKS	TIME (SEC)	RESISTANCE (ON BIKE AT 110RPM)
sprint	6	7.5% body weight
rest	60	0% body weight
sprint	6	7.5% body weight
rest	60	0% body weight
sprint	6	7.5% body weight
rest	60	0% body weight
sprint	6	7.5% body weight
rest	60	0% body weight
sprint	6	7.5% body weight
rest	60	0% body weight
sprint	6	7.5% body weight
rest	60	0% body weight
sprint	6	7.5% body weight
rest	60	0% body weight

sprint	6	7.5% body weight
rest	60	0% body weight
sprint	6	7.5% body weight
rest	60	0% body weight
sprint	6	7.5% body weight

Long duration (intermediate)

ALL WEEKS	TIME (SEC)	RESISTANCE (ON BIKE AT 110RPM)
sprint	30	7.5% body weight
rest	240	0% body weight
sprint	30	7.5% body weight
rest	240	0% body weight
sprint	30	7.5% body weight
rest	240	0% body weight
sprint	30	7.5% body weight

You would look to follow this protocol for at least four weeks. After that, the best way to alter the protocol is to add more resistance onto each sprint, that is, change the resistance from 7.5% to 8.5% and continue with the new protocol for at least another four weeks before considering changing the intensity again.

5

MYTHS AND MISCONCEPTIONS ABOUT EXERCISE

This book challenges one of the major misconceptions about exercise: that it takes a long time and you have to dedicate hours to it each week. High-intensity training means you only need to train for as little as 15 minutes and only a handful of days each week. However, despite the fact that this book has been written by two experienced scientists, and despite the fact that there has been substantial systematic research carried out that supports the benefits and effectiveness of high-intensity training, many people will refuse to believe that it works. There are people who would rather trust anecdotal evidence from their friends, advice that their PE teacher gave to them 20 years ago, or go with what they personally believe rather than current advice from science and health professionals. Exercise is a multi-billion pound industry that is built upon selling to the public: DVDs, supplements, exercise equipment, gym memberships and so on. All are designed to convince you that they are the only way to get fit and you need to spend your money on them. It is because of these attitudes that many people are not being as effective or successful with their fitness and health as they could be. With all of the misinformation about exercise it is not surprising that so many myths and misconceptions about fitness and training have arisen. We have already discredited the idea that you have to train for hours at a time to be fit and healthy. Now we will look at some other misconceptions that may be holding you back and put some myths under the scientific spotlight.

MYTH: YOU NEED TO HAVE A LONG AND THOROUGH WARM-UP BEFORE EXERCISING

Before exercising almost all of us will carry out some form of warm-up. The idea behind this is that it prepares us for activity by warming the body and increasing blood flow to the working muscles. If true, this should mean muscles are less stiff and there is less risk of injury. Generally, it is recommended that, depending on what you are doing, you start with a light jog or cycle and gradually increase the intensity until you feel ready to start exercising. Many exercise 'experts' will tell you that the longer and more gentle the warm-up the more beneficial it will be. However, do you even need to be doing a warm-up at all?

Surprisingly, research has shown that a warm-up can decrease as well as increase your performance. In studies looking at cyclists and runners it has been found that many actually take too long over their warm-up. This can mean that you have tired yourself out before even starting your exercise programme. One study found that cyclists produced more power before their warm-up than after it. If you cannot exercise as hard because you are tired you will not get the most benefit out of your training. At most you need five to ten minutes to warm up but in one research project they found that some speed skaters were warming up for two hours for a race that lasted just over 30 seconds! One of the main benefits of high-intensity training is that it does not take very long and the training benefits come from training at a maximal level. A long warm-up goes against both of these principles.

Despite the conventional wisdom that a warm-up improves performance and helps to prevent injury no study has convincingly shown that a warm-up protects you from injury or that a warm-up is even necessary. While there is no doubt that a warm-up raises your body temperature and makes muscles and tissues more flexible and malleable there is no evidence to suggest that warmer muscles perform better or are less prone to injury than colder ones. From an evolutionary perspective a warm-up also makes little or no sense. The gazelle that needs to warm up before running away from a lion is going to be that lion's next meal. If you have ever had a scare then you know exactly how fast your heart rate can increase and how quickly you can feel ready for action.

So, does this mean you should not warm up? Not necessarily, a warm-up does have some benefits. The most often overlooked benefit is the mental preparation a warm-up provides. A warm-up can help clear the mind and increase concentration. Many runners and cyclists often talk about being 'in the zone' and the need to focus on their training. High-intensity training is a strenuous activity and you need to be in the right frame of mind to be at your most effective. A warm-up can help you manage the transition from your everyday life, such as work and the kids, to the time you have set aside for exercise. The point to remember is not to overdo it. More is not better when it comes to a warm-up. Keep it short and do not tire yourself out before you even get going.

MYTH: STRETCHING BEFORE EXERCISING PREVENTS INJURY

For the majority of people, a pre-exercise routine also means going through a series of stretches and anyone who has taken part in a race will be familiar with the sight of people starting their run or cycle by 'limbering up'. Stretching generally consists of the simple, traditional poses, such as stretching out your quadriceps by touching your foot to your bottom or leaning over and touching your toes to stretch your hamstrings. Most people hold these stretches for 10 to 30 seconds, and this method is known as static stretching (holding with no movement). The reasoning behind stretching before exercise is that it will help to improve performance and, more importantly, prevent injury.

Stretching before exercise has been the focus of several research studies in both recreational exercisers, and amateur and professional athletes. These studies normally compare two groups over a substantial time period. One group does static stretching; the other group does not. The results are invariably the same. The injuries in both groups are nearly identical. Stretching neither prevents injury in the short or long term, nor does it increase injury. Whether you stretch or not will make no difference to you in your high-intensity training. Or will it?

While stretching has no impact on injury it may hinder rather than improve your performance. When you stretch you may activate the 'stretch reflex', an important protective mechanism for the muscles. Essentially, when a muscle is lengthened during stretching it has a threshold which, when it is passed, causes the muscle to contract, basically becoming tighter to protect itself from being stretched too far. If you stretch too far or too fast your muscles will tighten. Many of you will have experienced this as a quivering or sharp tug when you have been stretching. It is a bit like when your reflexes are tested by hitting your knee with a reflex hammer. This tightening actually prevents your muscles from producing as much power. Previous studies have shown that after stretching you cannot jump as high or sprint as fast.

So, stretching may actually be detrimental if you are undertaking a high-intensity training programme. Not only does static stretching not prevent injuries it can actually reduce your performance. If you really feel that you want to carry on stretching then you should use what is known as dynamic stretching, that is, moving your body in well-controlled motions. Rather than leaning over and touching your toes to stretch your hamstring you could swing your leg in a kicking motion. This type of stretching does not activate the stretch reflex in the same way as static stretching and it also teaches you control of your motions as well as helping to increase flexibility. If you do decide to try this, incorporate it slowly into your routine, rather than making sudden changes, and make sure the motions are well controlled at all times. If you are wildly swinging your arms and legs about you are more likely to hurt yourself or hit your training partner if they are standing too close!

MYTH: LOW-INTENSITY EXERCISE WILL BURN MORE FAT

For many people their main aim when exercising is to lose weight, more specifically to lose fat. It is no surprise then that people are always interested in which exercise burns the most fat. If you have ever been on a treadmill or an exercise bike you cannot help but have seen the 'fat burning zone' workout option. You have probably even tried it. These programmes have you working at a lower intensity with a lower heart rate. If the programme is called 'fat burning' surely it is the best way to burn fat and lose weight?

It is true that when you train at different intensities your body uses different types of fuel. At lower levels, for example, 50–60% of your maximal heart rate (the highest heart rate you could achieve when exercising at your upper limit), you rely more on body fat stores to fuel your exercise. At high levels, 70% or more, you begin to rely more on carbohydrates to fuel your activity. However, if want to maximise weight loss it isn't about what percentage of the energy used comes from each source that matters but how much energy is used overall. This is where the low-intensity myth breaks down.

If you were to go jogging for 30 minutes at 60–70% of your maximum heart rate you would burn about 150 Kcal depending on how much you weigh. About 60% of this will be from fat which is 90 Kcal. If you did the same 30-minute jog at 70–80% of your maximum heart rate you would burn about 200 Kcal. This time, only about 50% of the Kcal used would come from fat, but this is roughly 100 Kcal. This means that, although a greater percentage of the energy used at low-intensity exercise comes from fat, you will burn a greater amount of fat overall working at a high intensity.

Another reason why the low-intensity-burns-more-fat myth falls apart is that your body can for the most part convert macronutrients such as fat and carbohydrates from one form into another. A Kcal burned is a Kcal regardless of the fuel being used, no matter if it is fat or carbohydrate. Going back to our example then, the 30-minute jog at 60–70% of your maximum heart rate only burned about 150 Kcal. The 30-minute jog at 70–80% of your maximum heart rate burned about 200 Kcal. That is an increase in Kcal burned of 33%.

Exercising at a low intensity uses a greater percentage of fat, but working at a high intensity burns more fat in the same amount of time and more energy is used overall. Myths about 'fat burning zones' are mostly marketing gimmicks. They are trying to sell the idea to you that you do not need to make much of an effort to get fit or lose weight. This is why so many people become disappointed and disillusioned when their exercise does not have the impact they expect. They follow the advice given but they do not see any results. Losing weight is about how much energy you use compared to how much energy you consume, not about the source of that energy. High-intensity training is about working hard. The harder you work, the more energy you use and the more fat you burn.

MYTH: LACTIC ACID CAUSES PAIN AND FATIGUE

Lactic acid is considered by many to be the cause of muscle pain when exercising. They consider it a waste product that is created in the muscles as a result of exercise, most particularly because of a lack of oxygen reaching those muscles. The higher the intensity of the exercise, the more lactic acid is produced. Lactic acid has been blamed for the burning sensation during exercise and the sore muscles many people can have in the days following a hard exercise session. Overall, many people believe that lactic acid build-up hurts during exercise and that it is something that is harmful and counterproductive to both fitness and exercise.

Many gym instructors, coaches and personal trainers will confidently tell you that lactic acid is responsible for fatigue in all types of exercise. They will tell you that the build-up of lactic acid in the blood is the cause of exhaustion and that it is what stops you exercising further. Many of them will try to convince you to train at just below what is known as the 'lactic threshold', the point where lactic acid starts to build up. They are wrong. Lactic acid does build up during exercise but it is not the cause of fatigue. In fact, it is the exact opposite. Lactic acid is a fuel.

Lactic acid is not a waste product. It is produced in your muscles as part of the energy pathways that fuel activity. As you use up the glucose, you produce lactate, which is then used to obtain more energy. When working at high intensities it is what allows you to keep going. During this type of exercise it is the preferred source of fuel for the heart and brain. Lactate is also not just an important source of energy during maximal high-intensity exercise but also when working at lower intensities or when recovering from higher intensity exercise. This makes it essential for getting the most out of high-intensity training as you will need to use it to fuel your sprints and to increase the speed of your recovery.

The reason people who do more physical activity can perform longer and harder is not because they are able to withstand lactic acid or that their bodies produce less lactate. What happens is that, as you train, your muscles adapt to be able to more readily use this fuel source. This makes high-intensity training an ideal programme to help train your body to do this. The strenuous effort causes a greater production of lactic acid. This, combined with small rest periods that do not quite give your body enough time to replenish other fuel sources, forces your body to use alternative sources of energy more efficiently..

Finally, it is also a myth that lactic acid is responsible for the soreness of your muscles in the days that follow a hard training session. Even if you have not previously done any training all of the lactic acid will have gone from your muscles within a short time period, certainly no more than an hour. Muscle soreness does not happen until at least a day after exercise and often occurs two days later. The timing makes no sense for lactic acid to be the cause of this soreness and no research has ever linked the two together. Even though your legs may become sore during or after exercise, and although high-intensity training will exhaust you, it is not lactic acid that is causing this. Rather, it is what is allowing you to push harder and as you train your body will adapt to use it more efficiently.

MYTH: TRAINING NEEDS TO BE SPORT-SPECIFIC

A debate that has raged in sport for years is the notion of sport-specific training. This is the idea that your training should be appropriate for the activity for which you are training in order to get the most benefit and to see the greatest improvements in your fitness and performance. To be a good sprinter you should sprint; to be a good marathon runner you should run long distances. Essentially, you should train by doing what it is you want to train for. If this were the case, then high-intensity training would only be useful for runners or cyclists who compete in short sprint-based disciplines. As we have seen from the first chapter of this book this is not the case. The physiological changes that occur as a result of high-intensity training are applicable to both anaerobic and aerobic-based activities.

Perhaps you are training for the local rugby team and your friend is training for a boxing competition. You would both benefit from being faster and more agile, but neither of you would benefit if this came at the expense of a loss in strength or explosive power. Are these goals different? Do you and your friend need to train differently or are you basically looking for the same thing? Sport-specific training is a myth. There is no argument that there are skill-sets required for different sports that will benefit from training that simulates that sport (for example, dribbling and passing a ball, serving a tennis ball and so on). However, for most people their performance will be predominantly limited by their speed, power and endurance. Fundamentally, the best methods to develop speed, power and endurance are universal.

High-intensity training, while focused on short bursts of strenuous activity, stimulates many of the same reactions in your body that result in the beneficial effects that accrue with endurance activities such as long-distance running. At the same time, this type of training programme increases your ability to use lactic acid as a fuel and allows you to generate the larger amounts of power that are necessary in demanding bouts of activity such as the short, intensive sprints necessary in sports such as rugby and football.

While sport-specific training is largely a myth, person-specific training is something everyone needs to consider. What type of training is right for you? High-intensity training can give you many of the benefits of endurance or long-distance running and cycling. It can do this in a fraction of the time-investment as long as you are willing to put in the strenuous effort needed. Is this right for you? For some, the experience of long-distance training and the immersion in that environment is what they are looking for. They may find long runs a source of enjoyment or escapism. If this is you, then there is nothing wrong with these activities. Just make sure you are choosing them because the activity is right for you and not because of a misinformed view of sport-specificity.

MYTH: WEIGHT IS THE BEST INDICATOR OF HEALTH

Those involved in health and exercise are constantly being asked the question about what an ideal weight is or how much weight someone needs to lose to be healthy. As a nation we have become obsessed with weight, weight classifications and dieting. The media tells us that if we are 'overweight' then we are unhealthy and that we need to do something about it. Conversely, those who are thin are idolised and held up as examples of good health. We are told that we all need to be at our 'healthy weight' and many people will go to extremely unhealthy measures in order to get thin under the impression that they will be healthier just because they are lighter.

Obesity is undoubtedly a risk factor for several diseases and health problems, but how important is it? The truth is that the human body is incredibly complex. We do not fully understand how it all works but we do know that there are hundreds of factors influencing your health and fitness for both good and bad. One study showed that about one quarter of adults who were classified as having a 'normal weight' actually had indicators of poor health such as high cholesterol, high blood sugar and high blood pressure. The same study also found that more than half of adults classified as 'overweight' and one third of those classified as 'obese' had little or no indicators of poor health and had perfectly normal blood pressure and cholesterol levels.

So, why do many people believe that weight is the best indicator of their health? Part of the problem is our desire to oversimplify things. It is difficult to assess a person's health. It takes several different measures to really have a good idea of their state of wellbeing. We often need a quick indicator. One of the best known is Body Mass Index (BMI), a health measure we are all familiar with, based on the ratio of weight and height. This was developed by insurance companies who wanted a cheap and easy method of measuring people's health without having to pay for a lot of medical tests. The BMI measure also does not consider the composition of your body. Muscle is denser than fat and so weighs more. The fitter you are and the more muscle you have the less likely the BMI ratio is to give a proper indication of your health. Athletes often find themselves classified as extremely overweight or even obese on the BMI scale but you only have to look at them to know they are not overweight.

Quick indicators of health based on body weight such as the BMI have their place. However, we need to be aware of their limitations and to consider them in conjunction with other indicators of health and fitness. Low levels of physical activity, hip–waist ratio, alcohol consumption, smoking, poor nutrition and socio-economic factors also need to be considered. It is important to dispel the myth of healthy weight and re-evaluate our assumptions about someone's health based on their size. Big does not always mean unhealthy; thin does not always mean healthy. Weight is important but it is not the best indicator of health.

MYTH: EXERCISE IS SOMETHING FOR YOUNG PEOPLE

For many people the deterioration in health and fitness often associated with ageing seems inevitable. They believe that there is no point in exercising as they are going to get old anyway. They think that their diminishing fitness, strength and flexibility are natural consequences of old age. They have resigned themselves to a slow decline in both health and their ability to physically enjoy their life. For others who have never exercised it just seems too late. They feel too old to change their ways and there is no point in exercising. Despite a strong public health message encouraging the benefits of exercise for all ages and a general increase in activity levels in the older population, some people believe that older people should not exercise.

The reality is that the older you get the more important exercise actually becomes. Exercise allows you to remain healthy and retain your physical and mental abilities as you age. Regular activity lowers your risks of heart disease, diabetes and cancer, and lowers the incidence of Alzheimer's and dementia. Additionally, exercise can have other benefits and has been associated with increased social connections, a reduction in feelings of isolation and loneliness, and lower levels of depression. Exercise and other physical activity is essential for remaining healthy and feeling young, living longer, and having the energy to live a normal life and carry out day-to-day activities. Exercise is a major part of remaining in control of your life as you age.

What about the risks of exercise and the potential increase in your chance of injury from falling or other accidents? The fact is that regular physical activity helps to preserve muscular strength and retain bone mass. This helps to maintain your coordination and balance, thus actually reducing your risk of falling and injury. Being older does not mean you need rest or need to save your strength. If you remain inactive as you get older you are actually at greater risk of injury, hospitalisation, poor health and illness. As we age we cannot afford not to exercise.

Some people may feel discouraged by their current fitness, by chronic health conditions, or simply not knowing where to begin. What you need to remember is that exercise is just as effective for you when you get older as it is at a younger age. Your heart, respiratory system, muscles and joints will all respond to exercise regardless of your age. This means that much of the information that is available applies to you no matter what age you are. Also, while there are a few unique barriers to exercise due to ageing, there are also positive aspects. Retirement can be an opportunity to become more, rather than less, physically active as you now have the time to make exercise a regular part of every day. No matter what your age, state of health or your current physical ability, you can benefit from exercise. You can also begin exercising at any point in your life even if you have never exercised before.

CONCLUSION

High-intensity training contradicts much of the conventional wisdom of exercise and there are a number of sceptics who dispute the results of these training programmes. These sceptics are normally those who cling tightly to the myths of exercise such as the need for sport-specific training or the theory that lactic acid is the cause of fatigue. They are people who have normally invested a great deal of their own time training in their own way and they believe that to be a good runner you have to run, to be a good cyclist you have to cycle, and to be a good swimmer you have to swim. However, what may seem like commonsense ideas are often just the strongly held beliefs that have become ingrained in us due to constant repetition in the media. The human body is an immensely complex organism and one which we are only beginning to understand. Every day brings new advancements in sport and exercise science and in human physiology. You will gain nothing from holding on to entrenched beliefs that are often based on ideas and theories that are decades out of date. Many of us need to revisit what we believe about exercise, health and fitness. Ask yourself why it is you believe certain things, what facts are these based on and where that information came from? Try to keep an open mind and do not be afraid to discard your previous practices and try something new as you discover what does and does not work based both on the advancements in our scientific understanding of the human body and also on what works for you and what you enjoy.